1987

AIDS

edited by ROBERT EMMET LONG

THE REFERENCE SHELF

Volume 59 Number 3

THE H. W. WILSON COMPANY

New York   1987

THE REFERENCE SHELF

The books in this series contain reprints of articles, excerpts from books, and addresses on current issues and social trends in the United States and other countries. There are six separately bound numbers in each volume, all of which are generally published in the same calendar year. One number is a collection of recent speeches; each of the others is devoted to a single subject and gives background information and discussion from various points of view, concluding with a comprehensive bibliography. Books in the series may be purchased individually or on subscription.

Library of Congress Cataloging in Publication Data

Main entry under title:

AIDS.

(The Reference shelf ; v. 59, no. 3)
Reprinted from various sources.
Bibliography: p.
1. AIDS (Disease) I. Long, Robert Emmet.
II. Series. [DNLM: 1. Acquired Immunodeficiency
Syndrome—collected works. WD 308 A28732]
RC607.A26A3444 1987   616.9'792   87–10469
ISBN 0-8242-0751-3

Printed in the United States of America

CONTENTS

IV. The Future

PREFACE

Since the beginning of the 1980s, the phrase Acquired Immune Deficiency Syndrome has become part of the American vocabulary. AIDS is the most serious public health crisis in American medical history and it will be worsening in the time ahead. By the end of 1986, 35,000 cases of AIDS had been diagnosed, but they are merely the tip of an iceberg. Because individuals often do not want it known that they are AIDS victims, many cases are not reported. Moreover, for every case of AIDS there are many more of AIDS Related Complex, or ARC, illnesses associated with AIDS through a weakening of the immunological system that are not full cases of AIDS. Nor is AIDS an American health crisis only. AIDS cases are occurring increasingly in Europe and are reported in 74 countries worldwide. Central Africa particularly has been devastated by the disease. At present, there is no cure for the illness, and approximately half of those who contract it die.

In the U. S., the response to the AIDS crisis has been muddled by lack of clear and certain information. Approximately 70 percent of the victims have been homosexuals, and a homophobic response to the epidemic has intensified fear and panic. The result has frequently been that the AIDS victims are victimized again by public opinion. When the political commentator William F. Buckley wrote in an op-ed column in the *New York Times* that a way of dealing with the contagion might be to tattoo those with the AIDS virus in their systems, he raised a storm of protest from readers who were reminded of the tattooing of Jews in the Nazi concentration camps, citing the article as an illustration of an absolutist way of thinking that separates the "good" people from the scourged. A measured response to the crisis has been slow in evolving, and critics charge that the federal government itself has been reluctant to mount an adequate campaign against AIDS due to its association with homosexuality. In fact, heterosexuals are also at risk. Public health in general is imperiled.

This compilation concerns several aspects of the AIDS epidemic. The opening section concerns the status of the disease—what is presently known; how it is transmitted; how it acts on the body and brain; and what precautions can be taken. It includes the full text of the Surgeon General's Report, which informs the public about AIDS in candid language and calls for a campaign of AIDS education beginning in the nation's schools. Section II treats the disease and its victims, and reports on the medical efforts to conquer AIDS. Section III focuses on controversies that have arisen since AIDS was diagnosed in 1981. The final section examines the outlook for the future and includes a symposium of professionals in AIDS-related fields. Like the Surgeon General, the panelists point out that everyone, whatever their sexual preference, should protect themselves by restricting their sex lives. For the wise, they note, the "fast lane" is the wrong lane.

The editor is indebted to the authors and publishers who have granted permission to reprint the materials in this compilation. Special thanks are due to Ellen Morin and the Fulton Public Library staff and to the staff of Penfield Library, State University of New York at Oswego.

ROBERT EMMET LONG

April 1987

I. EXPLAINING AIDS

EDITOR'S INTRODUCTION

The spread of AIDS in this country and abroad has been covered in the media, but rumor and hysteria have often taken the place of basic information. This volume, therefore, begins with accurate and reliable accounts of what AIDS is, how it evolved, the manner in which it is spread, and what precautions can be taken to prevent infection. The first of these accounts, an excerpt from John Langone's article in the science magazine *Discover*, discusses the suspected origin of the disease in Africa and its route of transmission to the United States, and reveals how the virus enters the system and affects the body and brain.

It is appropriate that clear and forthright information should come from state and federal sources, two of which are included in this section. Reprinted in full is the text of the booklet *Acquired Immune Deficiency Syndrome: 100 Questions and Answers*, published by the New York State Department of Health. The booklet addresses many fundamental questions about AIDS, dispelling myths and separating fact from fiction. It is followed by the Surgeon General's Report, published in late 1986 by the U. S. Department of Health and Human Services and reproduced here in full. The thrust of the Surgeon General's Report is that in the absence of any cure for AIDS in the immediate future, a massive educational campaign must be undertaken. It should begin, he urges, in the nation's schools—even at the grammar school level.

AIDS: SPECIAL REPORT[1]

If you draw one cubic centimeter of blood—about enough to fill an eyedropper—from a person who's infected with the tena-

[1]Excerpt of an article by John Langone, *Discover* staffwriter. Reprinted by permission from *Discover*, 6:28–49. O. '85. © *Discover* magazine, December '85.

cious and widespread virus that causes hepatitis B, put it into a swimming pool containing 24,000 gallons of water, extract a cubic centimeter of water from the pool and inject it into a chimpanzee, there will be enough virus in the shot to infect the chimp. But if you put the same amount of blood from someone who's infected with the AIDS virus into the pool, if the chlorine in the water didn't kill the virus (which it almost certainly would), the virus wouldn't infect a chimp—or anyone else. Even if you diluted the virus in only a quart of water, the chances of giving a chimp AIDS with a one-cc shot of that water would be about one in ten.

Now that the AIDS epidemic has become a national obsession, it's unlikely that the preceding example will do much to offset the fear the virus has engendered. Nor, it seems, has the public's anxiety been assuaged by the repeated assertions of specialists that large quantities of the AIDS virus are needed to pass on the disease; that those quantities are transmitted only through blood and semen; and that it's highly improbable that exposure to toilet seats, drinking glasses, doorknobs, showers, or food touched by an AIDS victim, or to sneezes, coughs, saliva, tears, or sweat of a victim, will result in an infection.

America's irrational dread, a form of germ-phobia, is based on the notion that the AIDS virus is a super-agent resistant to everything that science can throw at it, an Andromeda strain with the transmission efficiency of the common cold. That's why 14 prospective jurors in Stamford, Conn. asked to be excused from a murder case after sheriff's deputies wearing rubber gloves escorted in the accused, who'd been diagnosed as having AIDS. That's why the only empty seat in a New York subway car recently was the one on which someone had spray-painted, "Did an AIDS patient sit here last?" That's why the Episcopal bishop of California issued a pastoral letter addressing parishioners' fear of drinking communion wine from a common cup.

There's homophobia, too, in the AIDS plague mentality. It's evident in the refusal to shake hands with gays, to be served by gay waiters, or, as happened during a city council election in New York, to accept a gay candidate's campaign literature. The homophobia has also served to confuse the issue of disease with that of gay rights; thus, when debate in the Massachusetts legislature over a homosexual rights bill digressed to how AIDS is spread, one lawmaker thundered, "I believe sodomy is a crime in this commonwealth. God didn't create Adam and Steve; He created Adam and Eve."

That bald statement mentions one thing that's of intense interest to researchers investigating the transmission of AIDS. Sodomy, in this case anal sex, is an alternative to vaginal intercourse, of which the best-seller *The Joy of Sex* observes, "This is something which nearly every couple tries once." It's also common practice among homosexuals.

Anal sex is an essential element in the AIDS story, and recognition of that fact has affirmed what researchers suspected when the deadly malady surfaced more than four years ago: AIDS is a blood-borne disease that in most cases strikes, and will continue to strike, homosexual and bisexual males who have been the receptive partners in anal sex, a practice that tears the delicate lining of the rectum and allows the AIDS virus easy entry into the body's circulatory system.

"It is unlikely that casual contact will play a significant role in transmission," specialists at the Centers for Disease Control (CDC) in Atlanta reported in September. "Current modes of transmission will remain stable, and sexual transmission of the virus will account for the vast majority of cases in the United States for many years to come. Homosexual men and persons who abuse intravenously administered drugs will remain at extraordinary risk for AIDS. The disease will probably become the major cause of death in these populations." (In New York City, 60 to 80 per cent of intravenous drug users, some of them homosexuals, reportedly have antibodies to the AIDS virus.)

But, as the fast-moving science of AIDS has sought to understand the workings of the disease, the researchers involved have spun for public a web of contradictions, misconceptions, and, occasionally, misleading statements that have been discernibly self-serving. Although heterosexual men and women who aren't intravenous drug users or recipients of blood or blood products still represent only about one per cent of U.S. AIDS cases, some scientists have made flimsy cases for the imminent spread of the disease into the heterosexual population. They've cited vague and unverifiable statistics about men who've contracted AIDS from female prostitutes, and made reference to the high incidence of the disease among purported heterosexuals in central Africa, while ignoring the likelihood that these AIDS victims have secretly indulged in socially scorned homosexual practices, used unsterile needles, or undergone ritual scarification and tattooing.

Adding to the scientific confusion is the rivalry between one AIDS virus discoverer, Robert Gallo, of the National Cancer Institute, and a team at the Institut Pasteur in Paris, which found its own version of the agent earlier. The French named their discovery LAV (for lymphadenopathy-associated virus, for the swollen lymph nodes that are an early symptom of AIDS).

When Gallo found his AIDS virus, he'd already uncovered two other viruses: HTLV-I, which causes an adult form of leukemia unusual in the U.S. but fairly common in southwestern Japan and the Caribbean basin; and HTLV-II, which was isolated from the blood of a patient with hairy cell leukemia but isn't yet known to cause the disease. In 1982, when reports of AIDS cases began pouring in to the CDC, Gallo speculated—opportunistic leap-frogging, one pathologist calls it—that the AIDS virus belonged to his family of HTLV viruses. When he isolated his own AIDS virus, it turned out to be remarkably similar to LAV, which itself was similar to, but clearly distinct from, the earlier HTLV specimens. Gallo called his finding HTLV-III.

Both Gallo and the French researchers think their viruses are virtually identical, but the French aren't comfortable with the way Gallo has extended his HTLV line. "Gallo was the father of HTLV-I and HTLV-II," Luc Montagnier, a member of the French team, says, "so it's natural that he should want the new virus to be a continuation of the same family." But Gallo's insistence on using his own designation has only added to the murkiness surrounding the disease.

Though AIDS research has been hindered by a number of scientific disputes like Gallo v. the French, much has been learned about the virus, and it's becoming clear that many of the original suppositions about its makeup, infective potential, and how it does its damage are invalid. Consider the question of whether the virus is really as powerful and as infectious as first believed. The answer seems to be no.

To say that AIDS is a weak virus isn't to make light of its wide range, the number of victims it has claimed, or its virulence. As of mid-October, AIDS had destroyed the immune systems of more than 14,000 adults in the U.S., leaving them defenseless against at least three types of cancer, or paving the way for the destruction of their lungs or brains. The number of victims is doubling every nine months. Perhaps as many as two million Americans suffer from a form of the disease called pre-AIDS (or have been exposed to AIDS and haven't yet shown—and perhaps never will show—symptoms of it). Moreover, AIDS is incurable and believed to be always fatal; more than half the victims have already died.

But it can also be said that the AIDS virus doesn't spread easily—not nearly so easily as, for example, tuberculosis, which can be borne on a cough; malaria, contracted from the bite of a mosquito; or cholera, spread by sewage-contaminated water or by food tainted with the feces of someone infected with the disease. As far as anyone knows, the AIDS virus is transmitted only through semen, during a sexual encounter violent enough to open a blood channel, either through mucous membranes or broken skin; through an exchange of blood that occurs when the needle of an infected person, usually a drug addict, is used by someone else; or through a blood transfusion from an infected person.

Thus, the virus's targets are highly selected and predictable. For men or women in the U.S. who are straight, who don't take drugs intravenously, and who aren't hemophiliacs requiring transfusions, the chances of contracting AIDS are less than one in a million. (The chances of dying in a car accident are about one in 5,000; of being murdered, one in 10,000; and of being struck by lightning, one in 600,000.)

Despite such reassuring statistics, the public retains its pervasive fear of AIDS. In an attempt to reduce that anxiety, we'll address a number of critical scientific questions about the disease. What does it do once it gains access to the body through an abrasion or a puncture? Can it kill directly, without relying on opportunistic infections to do the job, or even without knocking out the immune system? Can it attack cells other than the immunity-producing white blood cells for which it has long seemed to have a predilection? Is it a member of a family of human leukemia viruses, as most researchers suspected a year ago? Is there something special about semen, which harbors the virus, and about the rectum, into which semen is deposited during anal sex, that helps the virus to ravage the body so freely? Can the virus be transmitted, as gonorrhea is, to a woman through vaginal intercourse? To a man from an infected woman? Finally, where did AIDS come from?

Responses to these questions are replete with maybes, perhapses, possiblys, likelys, and unlikelys. Still, AIDS researchers now know enough about what the virus looks like and how it goes about its deadly work to enable them to give a few concrete answers, and to provide logical and well informed, though mildly speculative, responses to the rest of the questions.

The question of where the AIDS virus came from falls into the latter category. When the first half-dozen U.S. cases of AIDS were reported in Los Angeles in June of 1981, scientists at the CDC were convinced they were looking at a new disease—they'd never seen anything destroy an immune system so fast. Now they're beginning to change their minds: it appears that AIDS is new only to the Western world. Evidence is accumulating that the virus was present in Africa at least a decade before the first U.S. cases were detected, and is perhaps an evolutionary descendant of a virus that has existed in monkeys for as many as 50,000 years.

While scientists will probably never pinpoint the identity of the AIDS virus's immediate progenitor, they do know that AIDS is endemic in the central African nations of Zaire, Burundi, Uganda, Rwanda, Tanzania, and Kenya, and that a species of monkey plentiful in the area, the African green, carries a virus (STLV-III, for simian T-lymphotropic virus) that's remarkably similar to the HTLV-III AIDS virus. Scientists at the New England Primate Center in Southborough, Mass. discovered the simian virus when rhesus monkeys used for research began dying in their cages of a mysterious AIDS-like disease. While the scientists don't know how the virus got into the monkey colony, they've speculated on how it was spread: homosexual and heterosexual relations, as well as the spraying of urine, were common occurrences when the monkeys were caged in groups. (The incidence of the disease declined once the animals were housed separately.)

Unlike rhesus monkeys, African greens, which have passed along a hemorrhagic disease called Ebola Valley fever to humans, apparently don't get sick from STLV-III, probably because they've some as yet unidentified protective mechanism. But other species of monkeys do get sick from it, and in parts of Africa where many humans have developed AIDS or antibodies to AIDS—which indicates they've been exposed to these viruses—there's considerable contact between people and green monkeys. According to virologist Max Essex, who with Phyllis Kanki, a postdoctoral fellow at Harvard, found that one-half to two-thirds of the greens in the African AIDS belt are infected with the simian analogue of HTLV-III, the animals forage in garbage dumps and, when people try to chase them away, sometimes fight back by biting and scratching. Some Africans also eat the monkeys.

Such close contact with infected animals, some scientists think, was how the virus found its way into humans. Says Harvard pathologist William Haseltine, "All it takes is the transmission of one of those microbial parasites—viruses, worms, and the like—that's become well adapted to one of our relatives, in this case the green monkey. It gets into us, and we researchers see it in five to ten years. Bingo, that's it!"

Evidence that the AIDS virus existed in Africa before it struck in the U.S.—and that it required but a small mutation for the monkey virus to be able to infiltrate human cells—came first from researchers who worked in central Africa in the 1970s. One of them, Alexander Templeton, now a pathologist at Rush Presbyterian St. Luke's Medical Center in Chicago, was studying Kaposi's sarcoma, a skin cancer that accounted for up to 20 per cent of all cancers in some parts of Africa but was quite rare in the rest of the world. The cancer now is one of the three that frequently strike AIDS victims.

But that link with AIDS is, as far as anyone knows, only coincidence. The real importance of Kaposi's sarcoma in regard to AIDS is that it's evidence that an obscure and rarely lethal African disease could suddenly mutate and become virulent and widespread. Many researchers think AIDS has followed a similar pattern. Of the 600 Kaposi's patients Templeton studied, fewer than five per cent were afflicted with the most aggressive form of the disease, one that kills in a matter of months. Most suffered from a type that was sometimes disfiguring but rarely life-threatening.

Times have changed. The prevalent Kaposi's sarcoma in Africa these days is the usually fatal kind. Templeton has been astonished to hear from sources in northern Rhodesia that the incidence of the virulent form of the disease has quadrupled in the past 15 years, and is now responsible for 20 to 30 per cent of all cases of the malignancy.

Templeton speculates that the rapid spread of the deadlier form of Kaposi's sarcoma is proof that the AIDS virus mutated sometime after 1972 into a more savage form. The first real evidence for that came in March, in a report in *Science* by Gallo and an international team of collaborators. Studying frozen blood samples taken from 42,000 Ugandans between August 1972 and July 1973, Gallo analyzed 75 at random and found that nearly 65 per cent of the children and 48 per cent of the adults carried antibodies to the AIDS HTLV-III virus, which means they'd all been exposed to it.

Since there had been no outbreak of anything resembling AIDS in the years before the samples were taken, Gallo and others theorize that the virus must have mutated in the mid to late 1970s, roughly when it began to break out of Africa. Another reason AIDS may not have erupted into an epidemic until it came to the U.S. in the late '70s, Gallo says, is that Ugandans could have been infected with a virus just as potent as the current version, but for some reason were genetically resistant to it, and so able to harbor it without showing signs of serious disease.

How the AIDS virus got from Africa to the U.S. isn't known for sure, but it may have come by way of Haiti. During the mid-1970s, thousands of people participated in cultural exchanges between the French-speaking nations of Zaire and Haiti. AIDS then apparently was carried from Haiti to New York by homosexuals, for whom the island had become a popular vacation spot.

Precise knowledge of the origins of AIDS is less important to scientists attempting to develop treatments—and, ultimately, a vaccine—for the disease than a better understanding of the virus's makeup. Of special interest is how AIDS goes about killing off the very cells it should fear the most, the T-4 helper cells that serve as a master control for the body's immune response. Given the popular fear that the virus may begin infecting large numbers of heterosexuals, researchers are also focusing sharply on the access routes to the blood stream the disease favors, and the role, if any, that co-factors such as infection by other viruses, race, age, and blood type, play in the development of AIDS.

First, consider the AIDS virus, which, like all viruses, is a particle that inhabits a netherworld somewhere below what's classified as life. It's so tiny that it can't be seen with any optical microscope, and so sluggish in its natural state as to belie its vicious potential. Viruses are chemical packets consisting of a core of complex organic compounds, most often the nucleic acid DNA, surrounded by a protein coat. Almost inert outside a living cell and virtually devoid of any metabolic machinery, a virus becomes activated once it enters a cell of an animal, plant, or, in some cases, bacterium; fueled by the host cells' enzymes, it takes over the cell's equipment. Once a cell is infected with a virus's genetic information, which is simply a blueprint for making more viruses, its own genetic instructions are altered or blotted out by the new commands, and it may be changed enough to make copies of its new, flawed self, which can result in cancer. Or it may be forced to churn out many copies of the virus before eventually dying.

Ordinarily, viruses carry their genetic information in DNA, just as most other organisms do. But the AIDS virus is unlike most other disease viruses that affect humans. It's a retrovirus (HTLV-I and HTLV-II are also retroviruses), which means that it stores its genetic program in the nucleic acid RNA, and uses a special enzyme, reverse transcriptase, to make a DNA copy of its RNA program. This conversion enables the retrovirus to insinuate itself easily into DNA-formatted cells, turning them into factories for more viruses. But even among retroviruses AIDS is special, and it's these unique qualities that endow it with its deadliness and, perhaps, an Achilles heel.

The AIDS virus's distinctiveness isn't readily seen. Under electron microscope, the AIDS virus, unlike other viruses, which present a well defined shape, appears as a grainy smear, an innocuous-looking charcoal smudge about the size of the viruses that cause polio and the common cold. It's also susceptible to all sorts of outside assaults because of unique biological properties that allow its protein envelope to be easily eaten away. The AIDS virus, therefore, is unlike, for example, some viruses that cause central nervous system diseases, which are highly resistant to inactivation by heat, chemicals, and ultraviolet light. It thrives in a chilly environment, and heat de-activates it easily. If a sample suspended in a fluid-filled test-tube is left to stand at room temperature for 24 hours, it has only a ten per cent chance of surviving. Common detergents and cleansers—including hand soap—will kill it.

But the frailty of this virus outside the body can be misleading, for it only means that AIDS is vulnerable in the laboratory and on a surface of some kind. However, because of its dependence on and intimate association with certain of the body's cells, this virus is remarkably immune to drugs once it's inside a victim.

And once it gains entry, the unique composition of its envelope shows its insidious side.

For the past year, Haseltine has been probing the HTLV-I and III viruses, and he recently discovered that they share a peculiar biological property that enables them to reprogram a key component of a host cell's genetic machinery, altering it so that the virus's genetic information is read out far more efficiently than the cell's own genetic data when it's uninfected. This phenomenon, which speeds up virus growth enormously and isn't a property of most commonly studied retroviruses, is called TAT (transacting transcriptional regulation). The speculation is that besides allowing for efficient virus replication, TAT may also be the mechanism that alters the growth properties of the cell, causing it either to grow, as in HTLV-I leukemia infection, or to die, as in HTLV-III AIDS infection. The discovery of TAT is essential to understanding why viruses exert a dramatic effect on one sort of cell and not others, as appears to be the case with the AIDS virus.

For a virus to enter a cell, its specially tailored protein coat has to match receptors on the cell's surface. Some viruses, like the hepatitis A, that enter the body through contaminated food and water fit receptors on the epithelial cells lining the digestive tract. Flu viruses can be transmitted through food or by kissing because they, too, can lock onto epithelial cells. The T-4 cells, which the AIDS virus seems to favor, are processed in the thymus gland, pumped throughout the blood stream and serve as the master cells of the immune system. They aren't usually found in the upper digestive tract, a fact that makes the transmission of AIDS through contaminated food highly unlikely.

There appear to be sound, if speculative, reasons for the AIDS virus's affinity for T-4 cells. Half the genetic material in the virus's core resembles, in a general way, that of most other retroviruses that have been studied. The other half is arranged differently, and the size and location of the gene that codes for the shell of the virus is very different. Moreover, Haseltine has found that the virus can encode for at least two and possibly three proteins not commonly found in other retroviruses. What's now under investigation is which, if any, of these proteins is responsible for the unusual features of the AIDS virus, among them the TAT phenomenon and the fact that the virus seems to favor T-4 cells.

Once the AIDS virus, with its RNA translated to DNA, is inside the T-4 cell, it literally becomes part of its host, integrating its own DNA with that of the cell. It has the patience to evade the body's vigilant patrols of antibodies. Researchers and doctors who treat AIDS victims know that the virus can wait in a T-4 cell for weeks, months, even years (the latent period, or so-called carrier state, is generally two to five years) before it starts to destroy the immune system. If during this latent period some virus-infected T-4 cells find their way into another person, the disease can be transferred, even though the donor has few or no symptoms.

Eventually, the usurped T-4 cells, probably spurred by some other infection, begin to divide; this is the beginning of AIDS. As more and more T-4 cells are formed and come under the sway of the viral genes, they begin to turn out more particles of AIDS virus. The virus multiplies fairly slowly, reproducing itself about every twelve hours (the herpes virus, for example, doubles in half that time). Copies of the AIDS virus, at least in the laboratory, leave the cell calmly; each virus particle "buds" out of the cell, usually taking a piece of it along.

Despite the relative slowness of the process, the infected T-4 cells are eventually overwhelmed and die; with fewer of them left, the immune system fails. Originally, it was thought that only a small fraction of those infected with the AIDS virus would become ill, but now it's believed that more than 50 per cent will develop one or more of the symptoms associated with infection —destruction of the immune system, lymphoid interstitial pneumonitis, cancer, persistently swollen glands, and destruction of the brain, along with the serious motor, neurological, and psychological consequences that are a direct result of the brain infection. Once infected, a victim probably remains infected for life. The survival rate is unknown, but, given the percentage of AIDS victims who've already died, it's probably very low.

The drama that plays itself out in the body of an AIDS victim seems, at first, a straightforward one—a simple matter of a virus running wild through the body's defender cells, eventually killing them off and leaving the victim vulnerable to a host of opportunistic infections.

But the process of AIDS may not be quite like that. Increasingly, researchers are questioning whether this scenario is comprehensive enough to cover the broad spectrum of clinical problems associated with AIDS. Haseltine and others now refer to an HTLV-III epidemic, emphasizing that destruction of the immune system is but one of several lethal consequences of the infection. Sometimes, too, the signs of the disease—the various neurological disorders, the opportunistic infections, and the cancers—can occur in the absence of a severely depressed immune system. This is evidence, AIDS specialists now believe, that the virus is a lot more versatile than they once thought. "AIDS was defined for national reporting long before its etiology was understood," says CDC epidemiologist Harold Jaffe. "As a result, the definition was too narrow."

The virus's ability to destroy the brain is viewed as indicative of its versatility and perhaps of its affinity for cells other than T-4's. Evidence for that came in May at an international conference on AIDS in Atlanta. Jimmie Holland and Richard Price of New York's Memorial Sloan-Kettering Cancer Center reported that many of their AIDS patients seemed to develop a severe form of dementia that caused slurred speech, slowed movement, loss of memory, and psychosis.

Although AIDS researchers were aware that some of the neurological ills associated with the disease were caused by secondary infections such as toxoplasmosis, an inflammation of the brain caused by a parasite, or herpes, they couldn't explain why other AIDS patients had equally severe neurological problems in the absence of those infections. The mystery appeared solved with the publication in the September *Lancet* of a paper by researchers from the University of California at San Francisco. The principal author, virologist Jay Levy, reported that he'd isolated the AIDS virus from the cerebrospinal fluid and the brain tissues of homosexuals suffering from AIDS and its underlying neurological problems. Wrote Levy, "The results suggest that ARV [Levy's designation for a strain of AIDS virus he discovered soon after the French found LAV] could be the cause of the neurological syndromes in AIDS patients, and indicate that the virus can infect cells other than T-lymphocytes."

Neurologist Sid Houff of the National Institute of Neurological and Communicative Disorders and Stroke isn't surprised by Levy's finding. Forty per cent of all AIDS patients, he says, now suffer from some kind of neurological affliction. The most common is subacute encephalitis, an inflammation of brain cells caused by a virus, which, in severe cases, is marked by coma and death. Whether the AIDS virus kills cells other than T-4's in the brain disease cases is still not known. Houff says that T-4 cells would be the logical victims, because they're found in the brain as well as in other parts of the body. But, he adds, until more data are in, he refuses to rule out the possibility that other types of brain cells—such as glial cells, which support neurons and provide their nourishment, and macrophages, large white blood cells that devour bacteria and cellular debris—are also targets. His reasoning is that brain cells have many of the chemical markers found on the surface of lymphocytes, and these markers may be the ones most easily recognized by the AIDS virus.

The strong suggestion in Levy's data that the AIDS virus can infect and replicate in cells of the brain and cause neurological symptoms raises another question about the virus: Does it belong to the family of human leukemia viruses discovered by Gallo? Until a year ago, most researchers suspected it did. Now, however, after studying the virus's genetic material in greater detail, some argue that it appears to have far less in common with the HTLV viruses than with a subfamily of retroviruses known as lentiviruses. Even Gallo reported recently, "In spite of the similarities among HTLV-I, II, III, and bovine leukemia virus, the genome [all the genes in a set of chromosomes] is only distantly related to these other viruses. Instead, it shows greater homology to members of the lentivirus family."

Of the three lentiviruses known, one is responsible for brain infections in sheep (it appears to be closer in genetic makeup to the virus that causes AIDS than the AIDS virus is to the HTLV viruses), another for infectious anemia in horses, and the third for encephalitis in goats. Until the AIDS connection, says Houff, none of the lentiviruses was thought to cause disease in humans, and for that reason—and because they couldn't be readily transmitted to small laboratory animals for study—little is known about them. This much, however, is certain: when lentiviruses infect domestic animals, they become so lethal and unresponsive to drugs that the animals have to be slaughtered.

Although there appears to be a close structural similarity between AIDS and the lentiviruses, any attempt to compare their modes of transmission fails because of the lack of information about the latter. It's far easier to compare AIDS transmission to that of two other viral infections that are also prevalent among homosexuals, intravenous drug abusers, and patients receiving blood transfusions—hepatitis B and delta hepatitis, an unusual strain whose retrovirus was discovered only eight years ago.

Hepatitis B, with its 200 million carriers throughout the world, is far and away the most prevalent known viral infection of the blood stream. It causes a serious liver disorder and is believed to be the cause of liver cancer. Its annual attack rate on homosexuals is between 10 and 15 per cent.

Delta hepatitis, carried by a retrovirus with a surface coating of hepatitis B, can't function alone; it must either strike at the same time as hepatitis B or be superimposed on an underlying chronic hepatitis B infection. For a time, it didn't appear to be affecting many homosexuals. "But this picture is changing," says Dr. Jules Dienstag, a liver specialist at Massachusetts General Hospital. "Many doctors had felt that it was just a matter of time before this agent surfaced in the gay population, and a growing number of delta patients have been reported among homosexuals in Los Angeles. What worries us is that many gay men are chronically infected with hepatitis B. For the most part, these carriers have mild symptoms or none at all. A superimposed delta infection, however, could lead to acceleration of chronic liver disease or to fulminating hepatitis, which causes a massive destruction of liver cells."

A number of researchers have called hepatitis B, and now AIDS, venereal diseases, because they can be transmitted sexually. "It's as easily transmitted from a man to a woman as it is from a man to a man," Haseltine, in a minority view, says flatly of AIDS. "The virus is also now clearly transmitted from women to men, but not in large amounts, because not many women are infected yet. What remains unknown is the frequency of transmission that way. The fact that it occurs is absolutely clear at this point. There's no evidence to suggest that any kind of unusual sexual practice is required."

As authoritative as this statement seems, portions of it can be strongly disputed in light of epidemiological evidence and most of what else is known about how AIDS is communicated. A venereal disease is one that's typically and readily acquired through sexual intercourse or related means, and generally infects both sexes. Gonorrhea, for example, can be passed on not only through intercourse but also by heavy petting that involves the juxtaposition of genitals without penetration. Herpes, the only significant venereal disease caused by a virus, can be transferred from cold sores on the lips to the genitals by the simple touch of a finger. Chancroids—common, localized venereal ulcerations—have been known to occur on the hands of hospital attendants who treat them. But AIDS must enter the blood stream to infect.

"The most efficient way to transmit hepatitis B and, presumably, AIDS is to mainline infected blood directly into a recipient, whether by blood transfusion or a needle stick," says infections specialist Martin Favero of the CDC. The evidence for such direct blood transmission of AIDS is clear. Shared, dirty needles are responsible for infecting enormous numbers of drug addicts, who represent about 16 per cent of the AIDS cases—a percentage, it would seem, that could be all but eliminated by an aggressive public education campaign and liberalization of the laws prohibiting the sale of hypodermic needles. Between 80 and 90 per cent of severe hemophiliacs who regularly receive blood products are infected with AIDS (though less than one per cent are active AIDS patients), and so are many adults who received transfusions for other ills, and children, whose estimated rate for transfusion-associated AIDS is nearly five times that of adults. This situation should soon disappear as rigorous new controls over the blood supply take full effect.

Does AIDS' blood-borne route mean that it's not a venereal disease in the classic sense? The best answer, at least for now, is that it is VD, but only if one looks at those it most often affects—roughly 70 per cent of U.S. AIDS victims are homosexuals—and the *way* they engage in sexual intercourse. If it were a true venereal disease, far more people outside the high-risk group would have contracted it through heterosexual intercourse. But they haven't, and given the way AIDS is relayed, they're not likely to.

While some researchers claim that both the hepatitis B and AIDS viruses can get into the body through the surface membrane of the vagina—this has been shown in a few instances in animals—there's no solid evidence that it happens in people. And the AIDS virus has yet to turn up in vaginal secretions, which would be essential to widespread transmission of the disease from a woman to a man.

The conclusion, according to London venerealogist John Seale, must be that AIDS and hepatitis B are sexually transmissible diseases only in the sense that they can be transmitted by anal intercourse. "Blood is the only vehicle for transmitting these viruses," Seale says, "and chance abrasions of skin or mucosa are the sole portals of entry." In that respect, Seale concludes, both viruses may be similar to the common wart virus, which is spread from one person to another through abrasions of the skin.

Even *The Joy of Sex*, which bills itself as the "Cordon Bleu Guide to Lovemaking," sees danger in anal sex: "Unlike almost any other common sex practice, this one does have drawbacks. Usually the first try is painful, and while this may go away with practice, it certainly won't if you have hemorrhoids; it can cause injury, as the area wasn't designed for that, and extreme gentleness on the man's part is needed—anal rape, even of a willing victim, is accordingly out."

Anatomical drawings of the rectum and vagina show clearly why the rectum is far more susceptible to a blood-carried infection like AIDS. The inside of the vagina is made up of multiple layers of squamous cells that provide a fairly effective armor against infective agents. Also, heterosexual intercourse doesn't usually rupture the thick vaginal walls to allow a virus like AIDS easy access to the blood stream.

The inside of the rectum is another story. It's lined with columnar cells, which are more easily damaged and invaded by infective agents. Also, the rectum is more susceptible to tiny abrasions because it, like the rest of the digestive tract, is rich in blood capillaries that absorb nutrients from food. Thrusting an erect penis into the rectum, even after using a lubricant, can devastate the cellular layer, opening enough tears to allow easy passage of a virus in ejaculated semen to enter the blood stream.

That saliva is occasionally used as a lubricant in anal intercourse compounds the risk. "With our identification of HTLV-III in saliva, we propose that this might be a second route of transmission of the virus during anal intercourse," hematologist Jerome Groopman of New England Deaconess Hospital in Boston reported recently. Other practices involving the anus have also undoubtedly contributed to the AIDS outbreak among homosexuals. Fisting, for example, is an extremely dangerous and fairly rare homosexual activity in which first heavily greased fingers, then a fist are inserted into the rectum; the trauma is severe, as blood vessels rupture and tiny cuts are made in the rectal lining by fingernails. Dildos, or artificial penises, can, like fisting, prepare the way for an AIDS infection if a rectum damaged by them is then subjected to anal intercourse. Hemorrhoids, which plague many homosexuals and may be caused by the repeated insertion of an object into the anus, are blood-swollen capillaries in the lower area of the rectum; when they rupture and bleed, as they often do, the AIDS virus has a pathway in. Even the seemingly precautionary practice of douching before anal sex is dangerous, because it kills off protective bacteria in the anus.

While the receptive partner in anal sex is generally considered to be at greater risk, some specialists warn that anal intercourse is a two-way street. "Let's get rid of this misconception once and for all," says gastroenterologist Donald Kotler of St. Luke's–Roosevelt Hospital in New York. "The active partner in anal sex also stands a good chance of catching the disease." The penis, says Kotler, is fragile. Unlike the vagina, which has layer upon layer of lubricated cells built to withstand scraping, the urethra of the penis is coated with a delicate layer of mucosal cells that are easily invaded during anal sex. "It's pretty well established that the active partner in anal sex could transmit the AIDS virus if he were to abrade the rectum of his partner," Kotler says, "but you've also got to look at what his partner may be doing to him. If the passive partner were to bleed from the rectum onto the penis of the man doing the entering, then the active partner could have just as good a chance of contracting AIDS."

Beyond the fact that lesions in the rectum enhance the chances of AIDS infection, says Kotler, anal sex appears in a more subtle way to be an extraordinarily efficient means of spreading the disease. This is because of the types of immune cells found in the rectum and the variety of viruses that live in them. The colon, says Kotler, "is a filthy environment that needs constant surveillance from immune cells to keep foreign stuff out of the body." The most common cells found in the colon are B-lymphocytes, but T-lymphocytes, including T-4s, are also present. B-lymphocytes, Kotler says, are the favorite targets of the Epstein-Barr virus (EBV), a member of the herpes family, usually benign but capable of causing mononucleosis and cancer of the lining of the nasal passages, and Burkitt's lymphoma, an aggressive cancer of white blood cells that affects mostly children. Everyone is exposed to EBV at some time in his life, usually through kissing, since it lives in the cells of the throat, and when one is once exposed he harbors it forever within the B-cells. Kotler recently found that EBV is present in the mucosal B-cells of the rectum. The implications for AIDS are significant, because EBV is thought to be a co-factor in the development of many cases of AIDS, and at least one study has shown that before the AIDS virus can infect B-lymphocytes growing in a laboratory, it needs to be paired with an EBV virus.

The finding might mean that a recipient's risk of contracting AIDS would be greater if cells infected with EBV virus were already present in his rectum. The person doing the entering would also be at risk, says Kotler, if his blood already carried the AIDS virus and his penis were to pick up the EBV-infected cells from his partner's rectum.

There's yet another hypothesis involving the role of semen in AIDS. Says Essex, "It's likely that, in semen, the degree to which the virus is transmitted is related to some extent to how many lymphocytes are there, and there are likely to be a lot if the male is infected with something like syphilis or gonorrhea." Nongnuj Tanphaichitr, director of the andrology unit (the study of males) at Boston's Beth Israel Hospital, says, "When you have such infections, the production of white blood cells would be stimulated, and through some kind of leakage, they'd go out into the semen. There would be more in semen than in saliva, and they'd survive better in semen because of various nutrients—fructose, for example—that are there. Semen is also a survivor itself—you can set it out at room temperature, and it would probably survive for a day or so." Thus, another infection in an AIDS-susceptible or AIDS-exposed person increases his risk both of contracting the full-blown disease and of passing it along, especially if the receptive partner has a lot of T-4 cells clustered near the rectum.

AIDS may also be passed along during oral sex if infected semen is ejaculated into the mouth. It's not the virus making its way into the intestinal tract that poses the risk—presumably it would be inactivated in the stomach by bacterial enzymes—but its getting into lesions in the mouth, such as sores or bleeding gums. A person fighting a gum infection or flu is more at risk, apparently because in such circumstances the lungs normally shed T-4 cells into the mouth to help fight the infection.

The affinity of the AIDS virus for specific cells and little else means that under normal circumstances—and the experts emphasize normal—the virus probably isn't transmitted from person to person through contaminated saliva or tears. "Nobody can give you an absolute guarantee that one out of a hundred thousand times someone isn't going to transmit it on a drinking glass or through sweat," says Haseltine. "All we can say, and all we should say, is that so far, to our knowledge, it hasn't happened." Immunologist Paula Strickland of the Bureau of Laboratories for the District of Columbia points out that the AIDS virus is found in extremely small numbers in tears and saliva. As for parents afraid that their children might be exposed to the AIDS virus through a school cafeteria worker or an infected classmate, microbiologist James Thomas, chief of the bureau, says he would be concerned only if the children were engaged in some sort of direct blood-to-blood contact—such as a wrist-to-wrist blood-brother exchange. Says Michael Gottlieb, an immunologist at the UCLA Medical Center, "There's absolutely no evidence that it can be spread by a cough or a sneeze or by shaking hands with a person with the disease who has no open sores. In my clinical practice in AIDS over four years, I've been referred a number of patients in the no-apparent-risk category. Doctors wondered where they were exposed to the virus. In virtually all those cases, when a thorough medical history is taken over a period of weeks, a risk factor related to sexual activity or blood product recipient becomes apparent."

ACQUIRED IMMUNE DEFICIENCY SYNDROME: 100 QUESTIONS AND ANSWERS[2]

---

1. What is AIDS?

Acquired immune deficiency syndrome (AIDS) is a disease complex characterized by a collapse of the body's natural immunity against disease. Because of this failure of the immune system, patients with AIDS are vulnerable to one or more unusual infections or cancers that usually pose no threat to a person whose immune system is working normally.

2. What causes AIDS?

[2]Reprint of booklet, Nov. '86. Reprinted by permission from the New York State Department of Health. Copyright © 1986 by the New York State Department of Health.

Investigators have discovered a virus that is linked with AIDS. An international committee of scientists recently designated the virus as human immunodeficiency virus (HIV); it previously had been called human T-lymphotropic virus, type III (HTLV-III), lymphadenopathy associated virus (LAV), or AIDS-related virus (ARV). Infection with this virus does not always lead to AIDS, and researchers are investigating whether other co-factors may be necessary to trigger the disease. Most HIV infected persons remain in good health; others develop illness varying in severity from mild to extremely serious.

AIDS Risk Groups

3. **Who is at risk for AIDS?**

Approximately 95 percent of AIDS cases in New York State have occurred among the following groups of people:

54%—homosexual or bisexual men;

36%—male and female IV drug users;

1%—persons with hemophilia or others who received transfusions of infected blood or blood products (testing of blood supplies for HIV antibodies was initiated in mid-1985 to reduce this risk);

2%—female sexual contacts of men with AIDS or at risk for AIDS;

2%—children who acquired AIDS at birth from infected mothers.

Some 5% of AIDS cases cannot be assigned to these risk groups, but researchers believe that transmission occurred in similar ways. Some patients die before complete histories can be taken; others refuse to be interviewed.

4. **Why have Haitians been removed from the AIDS risk groups?**

Haitians were removed as a distinct risk group for AIDS when it became apparent that cases among Haitians were linked with the same risk behaviors as other cases—sexual contact, sharing needles, and transfusion of contaminated blood.

AIDS Transmission

5. **How contagious is AIDS?**

Unlike most transmissible diseases—colds, flu, measles, etc.—AIDS is not transmitted through sneezing, coughing, eating or drinking from common utensils, or merely being around an infected person. After six years of experience it is evident that casual contact with AIDS patients does not place others at risk. No cases have been found where AIDS has been transmitted through casual (non-sexual) contact with a household member, relative, co-worker or friend.

6. How is AIDS transmitted?

AIDS is not an easily transmissible disease. All evidence indicates that AIDS is spread through direct blood-to-blood or semen-to-blood contact. There is no evidence that AIDS can be transmitted through air, water, food or casual body contact.

7. Why are homosexual and bisexual males at high risk for AIDS?

Cases of AIDS among homosexual and bisexual males are associated with sexual contact, specifically anal intercourse and other sexual practices which may result in semen-to-blood or blood-to-blood contact. Anyone who engages in such practices is at increased risk for AIDS, whether they are homosexual or heterosexual.

8. Why are IV drug abusers at increased risk for AIDS?

IV drug abusers often share needles and other equipment for drug injection which can result in small amounts of blood from an infected person being injected into the bloodstream of the next user.

9. Why are hemophiliacs at increased risk for AIDS?

Hemophiliacs receive frequent transfusions of blood plasma concentrates which must be prepared from several hundred to thousands of donations. Cases of AIDS among hemophiliacs have been linked with receipt of blood products from HIV infected donors. Efforts are underway to produce synthetic clotting concentrates which would eliminate the risk of AIDS, hepatitis and other diseases that can be transmitted through blood products. In the meantime, heat treatment of blood components has effectively inactivated such viral agents.

10. Is AIDS passed by kissing?

HIV virus has been found in the saliva of some AIDS patients, but there is not a single case of AIDS that is known or suspected of being transmitted by kissing. If AIDS were transmitted by kissing many family members of persons with AIDS would be expected to have HIV infection. This has not occurred.

11. Why is anal intercourse linked with the transmission of AIDS?

The lining of the rectum is thin and easily torn. Anal intercourse can therefore result in direct semen-to-blood exchange.

12. Can AIDS be transmitted through oral/genital sex?

It has not yet been established whether oral/genital sex transmits the disease, but any activity which may result in semen-to-blood exchange presumably can transmit HIV infection.

13. Can AIDS be transmitted through vaginal intercourse?

A growing number of AIDS cases have been transmitted from infected males to females through vaginal intercourse. There are only a handful of AIDS cases transmitted sexually from women to men, although the HIV virus has been found in vaginal fluid. The very small number of such cases reported so far confirms that female-to-male transmission of the virus is difficult.

14. How do women get AIDS?

The majority of women with AIDS have a history of IV drug abuse, and presumably contracted the virus through sharing unclean needles. About 20 percent of women with AIDS have become infected through sexual contact with a man who has AIDS or is positive for HIV.

15. Does promiscuous sexual contact increase the risk of AIDS?

Promiscuous sexual contact increases the risk of coming into contact with someone who is infected with the HIV virus, as well as other sexually transmitted diseases, including syphilis, gonorrhea and herpes. All men and women are advised to know the sexual history and health status of sexual partners and to avoid anonymous, promiscuous sexual contact.

16. Can female prostitutes spread AIDS?

Prostitutes are likely carriers of HIV virus since they are often IV drug abusers. So far, there are very few cases of female-to-male transmission of the virus, but anyone who engages in sex with an anonymous partner is increasing the risk of contracting AIDS and sexually transmissible diseases.

17. Can use of a condom during sex reduce the risk of AIDS?

Use of a condom during sex can reduce the risk of AIDS since it minimizes direct contact with semen, a body fluid known to carry the HIV virus in infected persons. Since condoms are not failsafe, people should not rely on them as their only defense against

AIDS. All sexually active people are advised to refrain from sexual contact with persons whose history and health status are unknown.

18. Can use of spermicides reduce the risk of AIDS?

Laboratory studies show evidence that the active ingredient in spermicides (nonoxynol-9) inactivates the HIV virus as well as a variety of sexually transmitted diseases. Use of spermicides with condoms may further reduce the risk of disease.

19. Can a person with no symptoms transmit the AIDS virus through sexual contact?

Yes. Most HIV infected people have no symptoms and are not even aware they are infected. Any infected person may transmit the virus to another person through direct blood-to-blood or semen-to-blood contact.

20. How can people reduce their risk of getting AIDS through sexual contact?

All sexually active people—males and females, homosexuals and heterosexuals—are advised to limit the number of sexual partners and to avoid sexual contact with anyone whose past history and health status is unknown. Avoiding anal intercourse or other sexual practices which can result in blood-to-blood or semen-to-blood contact, and the use of condoms with spermicides should help to decrease the risk.

21. What is the risk of getting AIDS from a blood transfusion?

The risk of contracting AIDS through a blood transfusion has been significantly reduced through screening of all blood donations since early 1985 for antibodies to HIV and removal of blood found antibody positive from the transfusion pool. The risk of contracting AIDS through a blood transfusion was only about 1 in 1,000,000 prior to initiation of blood screening; the risk is now significantly lower.

22. Is there a danger of contracting AIDS from donating blood?

No. Blood banks and other blood collection centers use sterile equipment and disposable needles. The need for blood is always acute, and people who are not at increased risk for AIDS are urged to continue to donate blood as they have in the past.

23. Can you get AIDS by drinking from the same glass or eating from the same dishes as a person with AIDS?

Six years of experience indicates that AIDS is not transmitted in households where people may drink or eat from common dishes or utensils. The virus associated with AIDS does not survive well outside of the body and would be killed by normal washing of dishes and other eating utensils.

24. Can you get AIDS from public toilets, drinking fountains, restaurants, telephones or public transportation?

AIDS is not transmitted through the air, food or water, or by touching any object handled, touched or breathed on by an AIDS patient.

25. Can you get AIDS by touching someone who has it?

After six years of experience there is no indication that AIDS is spread through any form of casual contact, including handshakes, bumping together in crowds, contact sports, or even casual kissing.

26. Can AIDS be spread by swimming pools?

There are no cases of AIDS suspected of having been transmitted through swimming pools. The virus associated with AIDS would be killed by the chlorine used to disinfect swimming pools.

27. Can you get AIDS from trying on clothes in a department store?

AIDS is not transmitted through the air or by touching any object used or touched by a person with AIDS.

28. Can you get AIDS from handling money?

Years of experience indicates that AIDS is not transmitted through objects touched or handled by an AIDS patient.

29. Can you get AIDS from using someone's razor or toothbrush?

Since direct infusion of infected blood into your bloodstream transmits the HIV virus, it would be prudent to avoid sharing instruments that may come into contact with blood through nicks or cuts. There are to date no cases of AIDS linked with sharing razors or toothbrushes.

30. Can you get AIDS from dental instruments?

There are no cases of AIDS that have been linked with dental instruments, and the normal sterilization process would kill the HIV virus. Dentists are being advised to take special precautions to guard against cuts which could result in direct blood-to-blood exchange with a patient and potentially increase the risk of AIDS, Hepatitis B and other blood transmissible diseases.

31. **Can you get AIDS by being in the same house with an AIDS patient?**

No. Experts point out that no household member of any AIDS patient other than a sexual partner or an infant born to an infected mother has developed the disease.

32. **Can you get AIDS from a gay friend or co-worker?**

No. AIDS is not transmitted through casual contact. After six years of experience no cases of AIDS have developed among casual friends or co-workers of AIDS patients. There is no evidence that being around someone with AIDS, even for an extended period of time, puts you at risk for AIDS.

33. **What is the risk of living in a neighborhood that has a hospital or home for AIDS patients?**

None, since AIDS is not transmitted through the air or through casual contact.

34. **Can mosquitos transmit AIDS?**

A virus similar to HIV has been found in Africa in some insects, including mosquitos. There is no evidence, however, that mosquitos, other insects or rodents play any role in the transmission of AIDS to humans.

35. **Are people at increased risk for AIDS because they live in certain geographic areas (such as San Francisco or New York City)?**

People are only at risk for AIDS if they engage in high risk activities—sexual contact involving blood-to-blood or semen-to-blood exchange, or sharing needles.

36. **Is AIDS spreading in prisons?**

A number of prisoners have developed AIDS, but there is no apparent spread of the disease within the prison system. Nearly all prisoners with AIDS had engaged in risk behavior, usually IV drug abuse, prior to entering prison.

37. **Are health care workers or other occupational groups at special risk for AIDS?**

Safety protocols have been developed for health care workers and other occupational groups that may come into contact with body fluids of AIDS patients in their work. The federal Centers for Disease Control is following some 1,000 health care workers who have experienced blood-to-blood or blood-to-mucous membrane exposure to the body fluids of AIDS patients; many of these workers have had needlestick injuries while treating AIDS patients. There have been only three documented cases of health care workers (one in the U.S., one in England and one in France) who developed antibodies to the HIV virus after experiencing punctures with instruments containing the blood of AIDS patients. These cases demonstrate the need for health care workers to strictly follow safety guidelines when handling needles or other sharp instruments used in the care of AIDS patients.

AIDS Incidence

38. How many cases of AIDS have occurred so far?

In the U.S., there have been more than 26,500 cases of AIDS reported to the Centers for Disease Control over a six year period, with a steady increase each year since the identification of the disease in 1981. For an update of reported AIDS cases nationally, contact the Centers for Disease Control at (404) 329-3472.

39. What is the geographic distribution of reported AIDS cases?

Thirty-two percent of the cases in the U.S. are reported from New York State and about 23 percent from California. AIDS cases have been reported from 50 states, the District of Columbia, Puerto Rico and more than 35 other countries.

40. How many New York residents have developed AIDS?

More than 8,500 New Yorkers had been diagnosed with AIDS as of October 20, 1986. Nearly 90% of these cases have been reported from New York City. For up-to-date information on AIDS cases in New York, call the New York State Health Department at (518) 474-7354.

41. How many men have developed AIDS?

As of October 20, 1986, a total of 24,424 males have been diagnosed with AIDS in the U.S. Of that number, 31 percent are residents of New York State.

42. How many women have developed AIDS?

As of October 20, 1986, a total of 1,775 women in the U.S. have developed AIDS, 47 percent of whom are residents of New York State.

43. How many children have developed AIDS?

As of October 20, 1986, nearly 380 children have developed AIDS; about 40 percent of these children live in New York.

44. What is the ethnic breakdown of people with AIDS?

Nationally, 60% of persons diagnosed with AIDS are white, 24% are black, and 14% are Hispanic. In New York State, a higher proportion of AIDS cases linked with IV drug abuse have occurred among blacks (44%) and Hispanics (36%).

45. Is the incidence of AIDS increasing in New York State?

The number of AIDS cases is increasing each year in New York. In the first six months of 1983, an average of 82 cases per month was reported in New York State; during the same period in 1984, the monthly average was 142, and rose to 236 in 1985, and 269 per month in 1986.

46. How many AIDS patients have died?

Nationally, 14,755 adults and 222 children have died from AIDS as of October 20, 1986; about 5,100 New Yorkers have died from the disease.

47. Is the incidence of AIDS increasing among IV drug abusers?

New York State and nearby New Jersey have the highest number of AIDS cases among IV drug abusers in the nation. In 1985, approximately 37% of all New York State AIDS patients reported IV drug use; some of these persons also reported homosexual or bisexual activity. There has been a major increase in the proportion of IV drug related AIDS cases in the last few years, with a gradual decline in the percentage of new cases among homosexual males.

48. Is AIDS occurring only in our country?

AIDS is a world-wide phenomenon. In addition to the United States and Canada, AIDS has been reported in most European countries, African countries, the Caribbean, South America, Australia and several other places including the Middle East and Asia.

49. Do AIDS cases in other countries show the same risk factors as here?

In general, the same risk factors—blood-to-blood or semen-to-blood contact—are associated with AIDS everywhere. The specific groups of people affected by AIDS varies to some extent from country to country. For example, there are fewer drug abusers identified as AIDS victims in Europe, and more females have developed AIDS in Africa. Studies are underway to gain a better understanding of the similarities and differences of AIDS distribution in the U.S. and other countries.

Diagnosis and Treatment

50. **Is there a test for AIDS?**

There is no test to determine if a person has AIDS or will develop AIDS in the future. A test has been developed that can detect antibodies (substances produced in the blood to fight disease organisms) to the virus linked with AIDS. Presence of HIV antibodies in the bloodstream means that a person has been exposed to the virus and presumably is infected. A positive test does not mean the person will develop symptoms.

51. **How many people have been infected with the HIV virus linked with AIDS?**

Based on initial testing it is estimated that about 1 in every 3,500 persons may have been exposed to the HIV virus. Among high risk groups (sexually active homosexual and bisexual males and IV drug abusers) the rate of exposure to the virus may be as high as 1 in 3. This does not mean that all of these people are necessarily carriers of the virus or that they will eventually develop AIDS.

52. **What are the symptoms of HIV infection?**

Some people infected with the HIV virus have no symptoms at all, and may be unaware they carry the virus and can transmit it to others through sexual contact. Other people may develop mild, temporary symptoms which disappear after a few days or weeks following exposure. Some patients have persistent swollen lymph nodes without any other symptoms. Only about 5–20 percent of those infected by the virus develop the severe and fatal form of disease which is called AIDS. Symptoms of HIV infection may include:

—extreme tiredness, sometimes combined with headache, dizziness or lightheadedness;

—swollen glands in the neck, armpits or groin;

—continued fever or night sweats;

—weight loss of more than 10 pounds which is not due to dieting or increased physical activity;

—purple or discolored growths on the skin or the mucous membranes (inside the mouth, anus or nasal passages);

—heavy, continual dry cough that is not from smoking or that has lasted too long to be a cold or flu;

—continuing bouts of diarrhea;

—thrush, a thick whitish coating on the tongue or

in the throat which may be accompanied by sore throat;
—unexplained bleeding from any body opening or from growths on the skin or mucous membranes; bruising more easily than usual;
—progressive shortness of breath;
—forgetfulness, confusion, disorientation and other signs of mental deterioration.

53. What is ARC?

AIDS-Related Complex (ARC) is a name some doctors and scientists use to describe symptoms associated with HIV infection which do not fit the CDC definition for AIDS. Some individuals with ARC may die of their infection without ever developing full-blown AIDS. Only about 20–30% of people with ARC have so far gone on to develop the fatal symptoms of AIDS.

54. What is the incubation period for AIDS?

The onset of symptoms following infection with the HIV virus appears to range from a few weeks to many years. Antibodies to the virus seem to be present, and detectable in the blood-stream, within a few weeks of exposure.

55. What are some of the diseases affecting AIDS patients?

About 85 percent of the AIDS patients studied have had one or both of two rare diseases: Pneumocystis carinii pneumonia (PCP), a parasitic infection of the lungs which has symptoms similar to other forms of pneumonia; and/or a rare type of cancer known as Kaposi's sarcoma (KS) which usually occurs anywhere on the surface of the skin or in the mouth. In early stages, it may look like a bruise or blue-violet or brownish spot. About 30 percent of AIDS patients show symptoms of brain disease or severe damage to the spinal cord. AIDS patients also may develop unusually severe infections with yeast, cytomegalovirus, herpes virus, and parasites such as Toxoplasma or Cryptosporidia; milder infections with these organisms do not suggest immune deficiency.

56. How is AIDS treated?

A variety of drugs are being tried that show some promise of killing or inhibiting the activity of the HIV virus inside the body. No drugs are yet available that have been shown to cure AIDS, although the search for an effective treatment is being pursued vigorously. Most treatment is directed at the specific infections or cancers which attack HIV infected patients.

57. What percent of people have died from AIDS?

Approximately 50 percent of all persons diagnosed with AIDS have died. The death rate increases to nearly 70 percent two years after diagnosis.

58. Does anybody ever survive AIDS?

Some people with AIDS are still alive five years after diagnosis. Since there is no current treatment to reverse the damage to the immune system, we don't know how long AIDS patients can live.

59. Is there a vaccine to prevent AIDS?

There is currently no vaccine to protect a person from the HIV virus or AIDS. Researchers in the U.S. and other countries are working diligently to develop a vaccine. Scientists report that this may be difficult because the virus can alter its form in the human body.

60. What is the government doing to find a cure or treatment for AIDS?

New York State was the first state to appropriate tax dollars for AIDS research. So far, nearly $12 million in State funds have been provided to support AIDS research in New York State. The U.S. Department of Health and Human Services has provided nearly $440 million to fund research projects to find preventative and/or treatment methods for AIDS and/or the opportunistic infections associated with the disease.

AIDS in Children

61. How many children have AIDS?

Approximately 350 U.S. children have been reported as having AIDS as of October 1986. Most of these children, born in New York City, have mothers involved in IV drug abuse.

62. How do children get AIDS?

The majority of infected children acquired AIDS from their infected mothers, presumably through blood exchange in the uterus or during birth. A few children developed AIDS from blood transfusions prior to screening of the blood supplies.

63. How can children be protected from AIDS?

All high-risk women of childbearing age should learn if they have been exposed to the HIV virus, and should consider postponing pregnancy if they are positive. Women are considered high-risk if they have ever engaged in IV drug abuse or if they have ever had sexual contact with a known IV drug abuser, bisexual man or hemophiliac.

64. What is the risk of an infected mother passing the HIV virus to her baby?

Limited studies indicate that as many as 50% of infected mothers pass the virus to their babies. An infected mother can transmit the virus even if she herself has no symptoms of AIDS or ARC.

65. Can children develop AIDS from mother's milk?

There is one case of AIDS in Australia which may have been transmitted to an infant through mother's milk. So far, there are no cases of AIDS in the U.S. specifically linked with breastfeeding, but any woman who is positive for HIV antibodies is advised to refrain from nursing as a precautionary measure.

66. If a child has AIDS, can he/she pass it on to another child?

None of the identified cases of AIDS in the United States is known or suspected to have been transmitted from one child to another in the home, school, day-care or foster-care setting. Even baby twins, one infected and one not, sharing nipples, toys, food, bed and playpen have not passed the virus between them.

67. What risk does mixing with other children pose to a child with AIDS?

A child whose immune system is damaged by AIDS is highly susceptible to infections from other children in a school or day-care setting. Assessment of risk from attending school to an immunosuppressed child is best made by the child's physician who is aware of the child's immune status.

68. What precautions or guidelines should be introduced in schools to prevent exposure to blood or other bodily fluids from a child with AIDS?

All schools and day-care centers, regardless of whether children with AIDS are attending, should adopt routine safety procedures for handling blood or body fluids. Soiled surfaces should be promptly cleaned with a disinfectant, such as household bleach (diluted 1 part bleach to 10 parts water). Disposable towels or tissues should be used whenever possible, and mops should be rinsed in the disinfectant. Those who are cleaning should avoid exposure of open skin lesions or mucous membranes to blood or body fluids.

69. Is there a danger having teachers, cooks or other school personnel infected with AIDS?

No. AIDS is not spread through air, food, water or any form of casual contact. There are no cases of AIDS reported anywhere that are known or suspected of being transmitted through food preparation, use of common toilets or drinking fountains or merely having long-term casual contact with a person with AIDS. Therefore, teachers, cooks or other school personnel with AIDS who feel well enough to work would not represent a risk to students or other school personnel.

70. **Should there be HIV antibody testing for school children or school personnel?**

Screening of school children or teachers for HIV antibodies will not provide useful information upon which to base a public health policy, since those who are positive do not pose a risk to others in a school setting.

71. **If a child is bitten by another child with AIDS—what is the possibility of transmission?**

While HIV virus has been identified in saliva, there are no cases of AIDS known or suspected of having been transmitted through a bite. Transmission of the virus appears to require direct blood-to-blood or semen-to-blood contact.

72. **Suppose my child became a regular playmate of a child with AIDS?**

Casual contact, even over a long period of time, is not regarded as dangerous. In household studies no child in the family of an AIDS victim has been known to contract the disease through day-to-day activities or contact.

73. **What if my child is in a classroom with an AIDS patient who vomited or had diarrhea?**

Your child would be at no risk. Care should be taken to minimize direct exposure to bodily secretions or excretions from any ill person. Persons cleaning up such secretions are advised to wear gloves and to use a solution of household bleach and water (diluted 1 part bleach to 10 parts water) as a disinfectant. While these precautions are recommended, it should be noted that no cases of AIDS have ever been linked with exposure to urine, saliva, vomit or feces. The secretions linked with AIDS transmission are blood and semen which must enter the bloodstream of another person to transmit infection.

74. **Since AIDS is transmitted through blood contact, could a child get it through a schoolyard fight or during a contact sport like football?**

There is no evidence of AIDS transmission through a sports injury. The external contact with blood that might occur in a sports injury is very different from direct injection of blood into the bloodstream which occurs in a blood transfusion or in drug abuse needle sharing.

75. What is the State's recommendation on children with AIDS attending schools?

New York State has issued a recommendation to school districts that each case be evaluated on an individual basis. Decisions regarding the type of educational setting for children with AIDS or ARC should be based on the behavior, neurologic development and physical condition of the child. These evaluations should be made on an anonymous basis to protect the child against potential discrimination. The appropriate decision makers would include the child's parent or guardian, physician, public health personnel, and school officials.

Preventing the Spread of AIDS

76. What is being done to prevent the spread of AIDS?

A. **Education**: Since there is still no cure or vaccine for AIDS, education is the most effective prevention. Educational campaigns are directed to the general public and those in risk groups for AIDS, encouraging them to discontinue any practices which have been linked with the possible spread of AIDS.

• **All sexually active males and females** are advised to refrain from anonymous sexual contact with persons whose past history and current status is unknown, and to avoid anal intercourse or other sexual practices which can result in blood-to-blood or semen-to-blood exchange. Use of condoms can reduce direct exposure to body fluids, and reduce the risk of HIV infection and other sexually transmitted diseases.

• **Male homosexuals and bisexuals** who have had sexual contact with a number of partners are being advised to assume they have been exposed to the HIV virus and to refrain from sexual contact involving the exchange of body fluids. Use of condoms is strongly recommended to prevent contact with body fluids during any form of sexual contact.

• **Drug abusers** are being urged not to share needles or other drug injection equipment and to enter drug treatment programs to become drug free. IV drug abusers also should assume they are infected and use condoms to prevent spreading the virus to others through sexual contact.

• **High-risk women** who are engaging in IV drug abuse or who are sexual partners of IV drug abusers are being advised that if they are infected and become pregnant they can pass the virus to their child. The federal Centers for Disease Control has recommended that all high-risk women of childbearing age obtain voluntary, confidential HIV antibody testing to determine their health status prior to becoming pregnant.

B. **Safety protocols**: Occupational groups that may come into contact with AIDS patients are being instructed in safety precautions to prevent direct contact with blood and body fluids. Safety guidelines have been developed for: health care workers, dentists, laboratory personnel, ambulance personnel, funeral directors, prison personnel and others.

C. **Screening of blood**: All blood collected in the U.S. is now being tested for antibodies to HIV. Blood which tests positive is eliminated from the transfusion pool. Persons in high risk groups are being advised to refrain from donating blood. Sperm banks and organ banks have been advised by the Centers for Disease Control to test potential donors for HIV antibody and to not accept sperm or organ donations from individuals who are antibody positive.

D. **Anonymous, free HIV antibody testing** is provided by New York State for persons who wish to determine if they have been exposed to the virus linked with AIDS. Such testing is not recommended for members of the general public, but may be advisable for individuals in high risk groups so that they may learn their HIV antibody status and be counselled in behavior modifications to reduce further exposure to the virus and potential transmission to others.

77. How successful have educational efforts been in encouraging high risk persons to alter behaviors which can spread AIDS?

There has been a change in sexual practices among many male homosexuals, which is verified through a significant reduction in the incidence of rectal gonorrhea. Surveys of 500 homosexual and bisexual men conducted in San Francisco show that 81% of those polled were now in monogamous relationships or were remaining celibate. Moreover, only 36% of those surveyed reported that they had had recent sexual contact with more than one partner.

We have had less success in encouraging IV drug abusers to stop sharing needles, although surveys indicate that a significant proportion of drug abusers are aware of the risk of AIDS. Efforts are continuing to develop educational materials and outreach programs targeted toward this group.

78. What safety protocols have been developed for occupational groups?

All occupational groups that may come into direct contact with blood or semen in the course of their work are advised to take special precautions to guard against AIDS, Hepatitis B and other infectious agents. These include:

—wash hands following any contact with patient secretions;

—take special care in handling and disposing of used needles;

—guard against needle sticks, cuts and other injuries;

—notify supervisors of any direct exposure to blood, semen or other body fluids;

—wear protective clothing (gloves, gowns, and/or goggles) if direct exposure to blood or body fluids is likely.

79. How is the risk of spreading AIDS through blood transfusions being minimized?

All blood donated in the U.S. has been tested for antibodies to the HIV virus since May 15, 1985. Blood that tests positive is removed from the transfusion pool. The process involves use of an ELISA (enzyme-linked immunosorbent assay) screening test, with confirmation of positive results through a more specific antibody test known as the Western Blot.

80. How effective is the new blood screening test?

All studies indicate that the HIV antibody test is highly effective in eliminating blood from the donor pool that may be infected with HIV. In fact, the test errs on the side of "false-positive" readings, since only about 10 percent of blood that tests positive on the initial ELISA test is confirmed positive through a more specific Western Blot test. All blood that tests positive by the initial screening test is removed from the transfusion pool.

81. Are sperm banks and organ banks screening for AIDS?

The Centers for Disease Control has recommended that sperm and organ banks screen all donations for antibodies to HIV virus.

82. Is New York State offering HIV antibody testing?

Yes. A number of regional HIV antibody test sites have been established by the State Health Department to provide testing and counseling for persons who wish to know if they have been exposed to the virus. Testing is free of charge at these sites, and anonymity is maintained through use of a code system. Persons seeking the HIV antibody test need not give a name, address or any other potentially identifying information. Private physicians also can arrange for their patients to obtain testing. For information on HIV testing in New York City call (718) 485-8111; outside of New York City call (518) 473-0641.

83. Why doesn't New York State mandate testing of all persons for antibodies to HIV?

The State does not support mandated HIV antibody testing of any groups or individuals since the information is not useful in developing public health policies, but could be used to discriminate against individuals or groups. The presence of antibodies in the blood means only that the person has been exposed to the virus at some time. It does not necessarily mean that the individual is carrying the virus, is capable of transmitting it to others, or will develop symptoms of AIDS.

84. Why doesn't New York State isolate or quarantine persons with AIDS to prevent the spread of the disease?

Persons with AIDS or those with positive antibodies to HIV virus do not pose a risk to the public through casual contact. New York State takes the strong position that the civil rights of any individual or group should not be abridged by society without sufficient scientific evidence that it is necessary. All information accumulated during the past six years indicates that AIDS is spread only through direct blood-to-blood or semen-to-blood exchange, and not through the air, food or casual contact with persons with AIDS or articles they have handled or used.

85. Why doesn't New York State legalize the sale of hypodermic needles or dispense clean needles to drug addicts to prevent spread through that route?

The State is currently studying this issue to assess whether legalizing the sale of needles or dispensing clean needles will in fact reduce the risk of AIDS without increasing drug abuse. A current survey by the State Division of Substance Abuse Services indicates that 93% of IV drug abusers are aware of the dangers from IV use and are initiating efforts to obtain clean needles within the illegal trade. The most difficult problem continues to be the multiple use or sharing of needles in congregate settings.

86. **What is New York State doing to get accurate information to the public about AIDS?**

The State Health Department's AIDS Institute maintains a toll free hotline (1–800–462–1884), which provides up-to-date information about AIDS. The State also funds AIDS hotlines and educational activities conducted by eight regional AIDS task forces.

Pamphlets and brochures directed to the general public and to various risk groups have been developed and are being distributed through regional task forces, county health departments and various State agencies.

Educational forums are provided for occupational and community groups who have concerns related to AIDS.

Care for AIDS Patients

87. **What services are available to persons with AIDS or at risk for the disease?**

The New York State Health Department's AIDS Institute has provided nearly $15 million to provide direct services related to AIDS and to fund regional task forces and other community service organizations that provide educational and outreach services associated with AIDS. Services include:

—informational hotlines;
—educational materials and forums;
—free HIV testing and counseling;
—counseling for AIDS patients, families and those at risk for AIDS;
—assistance in locating medical, dental and other health services;
—transportation to medical care;
—assistance with insurance coverage, housing, civil rights issues.

88. **Where can persons concerned about AIDS get HIV antibody testing?**

Anonymous antibody testing is provided through the Department of Health's regional offices and some county health clinics for persons who wish to know if they have been exposed to the virus. The test is free and no names or addresses are exchanged. Persons receive counseling as to what the test results mean and preventive actions they may take to minimize further exposure to the virus or potential transmission to others. For information on the test call the nearest HIV hotline.

89. Where can AIDS patients get diagnosis and care?

Persons who are concerned about AIDS may contact the State-supported regional AIDS hotlines for the names of doctors who are familiar with the diagnosis and management of AIDS. Referrals are also provided for AIDS patients seeking dental care, psychiatric counseling, transportation to medical facilities, and social services.

90. Where are AIDS patients treated?

AIDS patients are treated in hospitals, physician's offices, clinics or other health care settings, just like any other patients. AIDS patients do not pose a risk to other patients or to health care workers who follow recommended safety precautions.

91. What is New York State doing to ensure that AIDS patients receive non-discriminatory, humane care?

The State Health Department has developed safety protocols for health care workers, and also assists hospitals and other medical facilities in developing in-service training programs for staff. The Health Department promptly investigates any complaints related to patient care at health care facilities, and will take enforcement action against any institution that discriminates against AIDS patients or does not provide appropriate, humane care.

92. Why doesn't New York State designate special hospitals and nursing homes to care for AIDS patients to ensure they receive appropriate care?

The State has taken a major new initiative to ensure that AIDS patients receive the necessary medical, social and psychological support services. The State Health Department has designated a number of AIDS Care Centers which are responsible for managing the total care package for a person with AIDS. Services include: inpatient and outpatient care, nursing home care, home health care, dentistry, psychological and social counseling, and, if need be, housing.

93. Who pays for treatment of AIDS patients?

Care for AIDS patients is paid for by the same means as all medical care; the government (Medicaid and Medicare), insurance companies and individuals. Most insurance policies cover AIDS medical treatment, although most have maximum allowances. The cost of care for an AIDS patient can range from $50,000 to $100,000.

Human Rights Issues

94. **What rights do AIDS patients have?**

They have the same rights as those accorded to any other ill member of our society. Unfortunately, discriminatory action has been taken against some AIDS patients by employers, landlords, neighbors, co-workers and others who are apparently acting out of unwarranted fears based on misinformation.

95. **Is it right to keep an AIDS patient's identity a secret?**

Since AIDS does not pose a risk to the general public there is no need for neighbors, shopkeepers, co-workers or others who may have casual contact with a person with AIDS to know. Discriminatory action has been taken against persons with AIDS by those who are misinformed about the disease.

96. **Can you be fired because you have AIDS?**

Some employers are reportedly discriminating against AIDS patients in spite of continued advice from public health officials that there is no reason to exclude AIDS patients from employment as long as they feel well enough to work. Persons who believe they are being discriminated against by employers may file complaints with the State Division for Human Rights at (212) 870-8400.

97. **Should insurance companies be allowed to require HIV antibody screening, and then deny coverage based on results?**

No. Since the medical significance of antibodies to HIV virus in the blood of a healthy person is not known, we do not recommend mandatory screening of any individuals or groups. There is a potential that discriminatory action may be taken based on positive test results. There is no direct evidence that an individual with antibodies to the virus will necessarily develop AIDS.

98. **Should people who have AIDS be banned from working in banks, restaurants, barber shops and other people-contact jobs?**

There have been no cases of AIDS that are suspected of having been transmitted through casual contact or through the air, food or water. If a person with AIDS is well enough to work, he/she should be allowed to do so.

99. **Can a hospital worker or ambulance personnel refuse to care for an AIDS patient?**

Health care workers who refuse to care for AIDS patients may be subject to firing and possible disciplinary action by the State. Hospitals and ambulance services have a responsibility to care for the sick, and to assemble a staff capable of carrying out that mission. There is a need for greater educational efforts to ensure that all health care workers understand the potential routes for transmission of AIDS and follow recommended safety precautions.

100. **Can funeral directors refuse to embalm victims of AIDS?**

The Public Health Law does not require a funeral director to accept the body of any deceased person. Embalming also is not required by law. The State Health Department believes that funeral directors, as licensed professionals, should take AIDS cases. The department has provided AIDS safety guidelines to funeral directors and embalmers, and most funeral establishments accept the remains of AIDS victims. Names of firms accepting AIDS victims are available through regional AIDS task forces.

How to Reduce the Risk of AIDS

Six years of experience with AIDS indicate that the disease is not transmitted from one person to another through any form of casual, non-intimate contact. There is very strong evidence that AIDS is transmitted through direct blood-to-blood or semen-to-blood exchange. Direct contact with other body fluids of an infected person also may increase the risk of AIDS, although no cases so far have been directly linked with other body secretions or excretions.

Based on this information, there are precautions that can be taken by the general public and by persons in special risk groups to eliminate or reduce the risk of contracting or spreading AIDS:

• Don't have sexual contact with any person whose past history and current health status is not known.

• Don't have sexual contact with multiple partners or with persons who have had multiple partners.

• Don't have sexual contact with persons known or suspected of having AIDS.

• Don't abuse intravenous (IV) drugs.

• Don't share needles or syringes.

• Don't have sexual contact with persons who abuse IV drugs.

• Use of a condom during sexual intercourse may decrease the risk of AIDS.

• Don't share toothbrushes, razors or other personal

implements that could become contaminated with blood.

• Health workers, laboratory personnel, funeral directors and others whose work may involve contact with body fluids should strictly follow recommended safety procedures to minimize exposure to AIDS, Hepatitis B and other diseases.

• Persons who are at increased risk for AIDS or who have positive HIV antibody test results should not donate blood, plasma, body organs, sperm or other tissue.

• Persons with positive HIV antibody test results should have regular medical checkups, and take special precautions against exchanging body fluids during sexual activity.

• Women who have positive HIV antibody test results should recognize that if they become pregnant their children are at increased risk for AIDS.

SURGEON GENERAL'S REPORT ON ACQUIRED IMMUNE DEFICIENCY SYNDROME[3]

Foreword

This is a report from the Surgeon General of the U.S. Public Health Service to the people of the United States on AIDS. Acquired Immune Deficiency Syndrome is an epidemic that has already killed thousands of people, mostly young, productive Americans. In addition to illness, disability, and death, AIDS has brought fear to the hearts of most Americans—fear of disease and fear of the unknown. Initial reporting of AIDS occurred in the United States, but AIDS and the spread of the AIDS virus is an international problem. This report focuses on prevention that could be applied in all countries.

My report will inform you about AIDS, how it is transmitted, the relative risks of infection and how to prevent it. It will help you understand your fears. Fear can be useful when it helps people avoid behavior that puts them at risk for AIDS. On the other hand, unreasonable fear can be as crippling as the disease itself.

[3]Reprint of Surgeon General's Report on Acquired Immune Deficiency Syndrome. Reprinted by permission of the U.S. Department of Health and Human Services 1986.

If you are participating in activities that could expose you to the AIDS virus, this report could save your life.

In preparing this report, I consulted with the best medical and scientific experts this country can offer. I met with leaders of organizations concerned with health, education, and other aspects of our society to gain their views of the problems associated with AIDS. The information in this report is current and timely.

This report was written personally by me to provide the necessary understanding of AIDS.

The vast majority of Americans are against illicit drugs. As a health officer I am opposed to the use of illicit drugs. As a practicing physician for more than forty years, I have seen the devastation that follows the use of illicit drugs—addiction, poor health, family disruption, emotional disturbances and death. I applaud the President's initiative to rid this nation of the curse of illicit drug use and addiction. The success of his initiative is critical to the health of the American people and will also help reduce the number of persons exposed to the AIDS virus.

Some Americans have difficulties in dealing with the subjects of sex, sexual practices, and alternate lifestyles. Many Americans are opposed to homosexuality, promiscuity of any kind, and prostitution. This report must deal with all of these issues, but does so with the intent that information and education can change individual behavior, since this is the primary way to stop the epidemic of AIDS. This report deals with the positive and negative consequences of activities and behaviors from a health and medical point of view.

Adolescents and pre-adolescents are those whose behavior we wish to especially influence because of their vulnerability when they are exploring their own sexuality (heterosexual and homosexual) and perhaps experimenting with drugs. Teenagers often consider themselves immortal, and these young people may be putting themselves at great risk.

Education about AIDS should start in early elementary school and at home so that children can grow up knowing the behavior to avoid to protect themselves from exposure to the AIDS virus. The threat of AIDS can provide an opportunity for parents to instill in their children their own moral and ethical standards.

Those of us who are parents, educators and community leaders, indeed all adults, cannot disregard this responsibility to educate our young. The need is critical and the price of neglect is high. The lives of our young people depend on our fulfilling our responsibility.

AIDS is an infectious disease. It is contagious, but it cannot be spread in the same manner as a common cold or measles or chicken pox. It is contagious in the same way that sexually transmitted diseases, such as syphilis and gonorrhea, are contagious. AIDS can also be spread through the sharing of intravenous drug needles and syringes used for injecting illicit drugs.

AIDS is *not* spread by common everyday contact but by sexual contact (penis-vagina, penis-rectum, mouth-rectum, mouth-vagina, mouth-penis). Yet there is great misunderstanding resulting in unfounded fear that AIDS can be spread by casual, non-sexual contact. The first cases of AIDS were reported in this country in 1981. We would know by now if AIDS were passed by casual, non-sexual contact.

Today those practicing high risk behavior who become infected with the AIDS virus are found mainly among homosexual and bisexual men and male and female intravenous drug users. Heterosexual transmission is expected to account for an increasing proportion of those who become infected with the AIDS virus in the future.

At the beginning of the AIDS epidemic many Americans had little sympathy for people with AIDS. The feeling was that somehow people from certain groups "deserved" their illness. Let us put those feelings behind us. We are fighting a disease, not people. Those who are already afflicted are sick people and need our care as do all sick patients. The country must face this epidemic as a unified society. We must prevent the spread of AIDS while at the same time preserving our humanity and intimacy.

AIDS is a life-threatening disease and a major public health issue. Its impact on our society is and will continue to be devastating. By the end of 1991, an estimated 270,000 cases of AIDS will have occurred with 179,000 deaths within the decade since the disease was first recognized. In the year 1991, an estimated 145,000 patients with AIDS will need health and supportive services at a total cost of between $8 and $16 billion. However, AIDS is preventable. It can be controlled by changes in personal behavior. It is the responsibility of every citizen to be informed about AIDS and to exercise the appropriate preventive measures. This report will tell you how.

The spread of AIDS can and must be stopped.
—C. Everett Koop, M.D., Sc.D.
Surgeon General

AIDS

AIDS CAUSED BY VIRUS

The letters A-I-D-S stand for Acquired Immune Deficiency Syndrome. When a person is sick with AIDS, he/she is in the final stages of a series of health problems caused by a virus (germ) that can be passed from one person to another chiefly during sexual contact or through the sharing of intravenous drug needles and syringes used for "shooting" drugs. Scientists have named the AIDS virus "HIV or HTLV-III or LAV."* These abbreviations stand for information denoting a virus that attacks white blood cells (T-Lymphocytes) in the human blood. Throughout this publication, we will call the virus the "AIDS virus." The AIDS virus attacks a person's immune system and damages his/her ability to fight other disease. Without a functioning immune system to ward off other germs, he/she now becomes vulnerable to becoming infected by bacteria, protozoa, fungi, and other viruses and malignancies, which may cause life-threatening illness, such as pneumonia, meningitis, and cancer.

NO KNOWN CURE

There is presently no cure for AIDS. There is presently no vaccine to prevent AIDS.

VIRUS INVADES BLOOD STREAM

When the AIDS virus enters the blood stream, it begins to attack certain white blood cells (T-Lymphocytes). Substances called antibodies are produced by the body. These antibodies can be detected in the blood by a simple test, usually two weeks to three months after infection. Even before the antibody test is positive, the victim can pass the virus to others by methods that will be explained.

---

*These are different names given to AIDS virus by the scientific community: HIV—Human Immunodeficiency Virus; HTLV-III—Human T-Lymphotropic Virus Type III; LAV—Lymphadenopathy Associated Virus.

Once an individual is infected, there are several possibilities. Some people may remain well but even so they are able to infect others. Others may develop a disease that is less serious than AIDS referred to as AIDS Related Complex (ARC). In some people the protective immune system may be destroyed by the virus and then other germs (bacteria, protozoa, fungi and other viruses) and cancers that ordinarily would never get a foothold cause "opportunistic diseases"—using the *opportunity* of lowered resistance to infect and destroy. Some of the most common are *Pneumocystis carinii* pneumonia and tuberculosis. Individuals infected with the AIDS virus may also develop certain types of cancers such as Kaposi's sarcoma. These infected people have classic AIDS. Evidence shows that the AIDS virus may also attack the nervous system, causing damage to the brain.

Signs and Symptoms

No Signs

Some people remain apparently well after infection with the AIDS virus. They may have no physically apparent symptoms of illness. However, if proper precautions are not used with sexual contacts and/or intravenous drug use, these infected individuals can spread the virus to others. Anyone who thinks he or she is infected or involved in high risk behaviors should not donate his/her blood, organs, tissues, or sperm because they may now contain the AIDS virus.

ARC

AIDS-Related Complex (ARC) is a condition caused by the AIDS virus in which the patient tests positive for AIDS infection and has a specific set of clinical symptoms. However, ARC patients' symptoms are often less severe than those with the disease we call classic AIDS. Signs and symptoms of ARC may include loss of appetite, weight loss, fever, night sweats, skin rashes, diarrhea, tiredness, lack of resistance to infection, or swollen lymph nodes. These are also signs and symptoms of many other diseases and a physician should be consulted.

AIDS

Only a qualified health professional can diagnose AIDS, which is the result of a natural progress of infection by the AIDS virus. AIDS destroys the body's immune (defense) system and allows otherwise controllable infections to invade the body and cause additional diseases. These opportunistic diseases would not otherwise gain a foothold in the body. These opportunistic diseases may eventually cause death.

Some symptoms and signs of AIDS and the "opportunistic infections" may include a persistent cough and fever associated with shortness of breath or difficult breathing and may be the symptoms of *Pneumocystis carinii* pneumonia. Multiple purplish blotches and bumps on the skin may be a sign of Kaposi's sarcoma. The AIDS virus in all infected people is essentially the same; the reactions of individuals may differ.

Long Term

The AIDS virus may also attack the nervous system and cause delayed damage to the brain. This damage may take years to develop and the symptoms may show up as memory loss, indifference, loss of coordination, partial paralysis, or mental disorder. These symptoms may occur alone, or with other symptoms mentioned earlier.

AIDS: The Present Situation

The number of people estimated to be infected with the AIDS virus in the United States is about 1.5 million. All of these individuals are assumed to be capable of spreading the virus sexually (heterosexually or homosexually) or by sharing needles and syringes or other implements for intravenous drug use. Of these, an estimated 100,000 to 200,000 will come down with AIDS Related Complex (ARC). It is difficult to predict the number who will develop ARC or AIDS because symptoms sometimes take as long as nine years to show up. With our present knowledge, scientists predict that 20 to 30 percent of those infected with the AIDS virus will develop an illness that fits an accepted definition of AIDS within five years. The number of persons known to have AIDS in the United States to date is over 25,000; of these, about half have died of the disease. Since there is no cure, the others are expected to also eventually die from their disease.

The majority of infected antibody positive individuals who carry the AIDS virus show no disease symptoms and may not come down with the disease for many years, if ever.

No Risk from Casual Contact

There is no known risk of non-sexual infection in most of the situations we encounter in our daily lives. We know that family members living with individuals who have the AIDS virus do not become infected except through sexual contact. There is no evidence of transmission (spread) of AIDS virus by everyday contact even though these family members shared food, towels, cups, razors, even toothbrushes, and kissed each other.

Health Workers

We know even more about health care workers exposed to AIDS patients. About 2,500 health workers who were caring for AIDS patients when they were sickest have been carefully studied and tested for infection with the AIDS virus. These doctors, nurses and other health care givers have been exposed to the AIDS patients' blood, stool and other body fluids. Approximately 750 of these health workers reported possible additional exposure by direct contact with a patient's body fluid through spills or being accidentally stuck with a needle. Upon testing these 750, only 3 who had accidentally stuck themselves with a needle had a positive antibody test for exposure to the AIDS virus. Because health workers had much more contact with patients and their body fluids than would be expected from common everyday contact, it is clear that the AIDS virus is not transmitted by casual contact.

Control of Certain Behaviors Can Stop Further Spread of AIDS

Knowing the facts about AIDS can prevent the spread of the disease. Education of those who risk infecting themselves or infecting other people is the only way we can stop the spread of AIDS. People must be responsible about their sexual behavior and must avoid the use of illicit intravenous drugs and needle sharing. We will describe the types of behavior that lead to infection by the AIDS virus and the personal measures that must be taken for effective protection. If we are to stop the AIDS epidemic, we all must understand the disease—its cause, its nature, and its prevention. *Precautions must be taken*. The AIDS virus infects persons who expose themselves to known risk behavior, such as certain types of homosexual and heterosexual activities or sharing intravenous drug equipment.

Risks

Although the initial discovery was in the homosexual community, AIDS is not a disease only of homosexuals. AIDS is found in heterosexual people as well. AIDS is not a black or white disease. AIDS is not just a male disease. AIDS is found in women; it is found in children. In the future AIDS will probably increase and spread among people who are not homosexual or intravenous drug abusers in the same manner as other sexually transmitted diseases like syphilis and gonorrhea.

Sex between Men

Men who have sexual relations with other men are especially at risk. About 70 percent of AIDS victims throughout the country are male homosexuals and bisexuals. This percentage probably will decline as heterosexual transmission increases. *Infection results from a sexual relationship with an infected person.*

Multiple Partners

The risk of infection increases according to the number of sexual partners one has, *male or female.* The more partners you have, the greater the risk of becoming infected with the AIDS virus.

How Exposed

Although the AIDS virus is found in several body fluids, a person acquires the virus during sexual contact with an infected person's blood or semen and possibly vaginal secretions. The virus then enters a person's blood stream through their rectum, vagina or penis.

Small (unseen by the naked eye) tears in the surface lining of the vagina or rectum may occur during insertion of the penis, fingers, or other objects, thus opening an avenue for entrance of the virus directly into the blood stream; therefore, the AIDS virus can be passed from penis to rectum and vagina and vice versa without a visible tear in the tissue or the presence of blood.

PREVENTION OF SEXUAL TRANSMISSION— KNOW YOUR PARTNER

Couples who maintain mutually faithful monogamous relationships (only one continuing sexual partner) are protected from AIDS through sexual transmission. If you have been faithful for at least five years and your partner has been faithful too, neither of you is at risk. If you have not been faithful, then you and your partner are at risk. If your partner has not been faithful, then your partner is at risk which also puts you at risk. This is true for both heterosexual and homosexual couples. Unless it is possible to know with *absolute certainty* that neither you nor your sexual partner is carrying the virus of AIDS, you must use protective behavior. *Absolute certainty* means not only that you and your partner have maintained a mutually faithful monogamous sexual relationship, but it means that neither you nor your partner has used illegal intravenous drugs.

AIDS: You Can Protect Yourself from Infection

Some personal measures are adequate to safely protect yourself and others from infection by the AIDS virus and its complications. Among these are:

• If you have been involved in any of the high risk sexual activities described above or have injected illicit intravenous drugs into your body, you should have a blood test to see if you have been infected with the AIDS virus.

• If your test is positive or if you engage in high risk activities and choose not to have a test, you should tell your sexual partner. If you jointly decide to have sex, you must protect your partner by always using a rubber (condom) during (start to finish) sexual intercourse (vagina or rectum).

• If your partner has a positive blood test showing that he/she has been infected with the AIDS virus or you suspect that he/she has been exposed by previous heterosexual or homosexual behavior or use of intravenous drugs with shared needles and syringes, a rubber (condom) should always be used during (start to finish) sexual intercourse (vagina or rectum).

• If you or your partner is at high risk, avoid mouth contact with the penis, vagina, or rectum.
• Avoid all sexual activities which could cause cuts or tears in the linings of the rectum, vagina, or penis.
• Single teen-age girls have been warned that pregnancy and contracting sexually transmitted diseases can be the result of only one act of sexual intercourse. They have been taught to say *NO* to sex! They have been taught to say *NO* to drugs! By saying *NO* to sex and drugs, they can avoid AIDS which can *kill* them! The same is true for teenage boys who should also not have rectal intercourse with other males. It may result in AIDS.
• Do not have sex with prostitutes. Infected male and female prostitutes are frequently also intravenous drug abusers; therefore, they may infect clients by sexual intercourse and other intravenous drug abusers by sharing their intravenous drug equipment. Female prostitutes also can infect their unborn babies.

INTRAVENOUS DRUG USERS

Drug abusers who inject drugs into their veins are another population group at high risk and with high rates of infection by the AIDS virus. Users of intravenous drugs make up 25 percent of the cases of AIDS throughout the country. The AIDS virus is carried in contaminated blood left in the needle, syringe, or other drug related implements and the virus is injected into the new victim by reusing dirty syringes and needles. Even the smallest amount of infected blood left in a used needle or syringe can contain live AIDS virus to be passed on to the next user of those dirty implements.

No one should shoot up drugs because addiction, poor health, family disruption, emotional disturbances and death could follow. However, many drug users are addicted to drugs and for one reason or another have not changed their behavior. For these people, the only way not to get AIDS is *to use a clean, previously unused* needle, syringe or any other implement necessary for the injection of the drug solution.

HEMOPHILIA

Some persons with hemophilia (a blood clotting disorder that makes them subject to bleeding) have been infected with the AIDS virus either through blood transfusion or the use of blood products that help their blood clot. Now that we know how to prepare safe blood products to aid clotting, this is unlikely to happen. This group represents a very small percentage of the cases of AIDS throughout the country.

BLOOD TRANSFUSION

Currently all blood donors are initially screened and blood is *not* accepted from high risk individuals. Blood that has been collected for use is tested for the presence of antibody to the AIDS virus. However, some people may have had a blood transfusion prior to March 1985 before we knew how to screen blood for safe transfusion and may have become infected with the AIDS virus. Fortunately there are not now a large number of these cases. With routine testing of blood products, the blood supply for transfusion is now safer that it has ever been with regard to AIDS.

Persons who have engaged in homosexual activities or have shot street drugs within the last 10 years should *never* donate blood.

MOTHER CAN INFECT NEWBORN

If a woman is infected with the AIDS virus and becomes pregnant, she is more likely to develop ARC or classic AIDS, and she can pass the AIDS virus to her unborn child. Approximately one third of the babies born to AIDS-infected mothers will also be infected with the AIDS virus. Most of the infected babies will eventually develop the disease and die. Several of these babies have been born to wives of hemophiliac men infected with the AIDS virus by way of contaminated blood products. Some babies have also been born to women who became infected with the AIDS virus by bisexual partners who had the virus. Almost all babies with AIDS have been born to women who were intravenous drug users or the sexual partners of intravenous drug users who were infected with the AIDS virus. More such babies can be expected.

Think carefully if you plan on becoming pregnant. If there is any chance that you may be in any high risk group or that you have had sex with someone in a high risk group, such as homosexual and bisexual males, drug abusers and their sexual partners, see your doctor.

SUMMARY

AIDS affects certain groups of the population. Homosexual and bisexual males who have had sexual contact with other homosexual or bisexual males as well as those who "shoot" street drugs are at greatest risk of exposure, infection and eventual death. Sexual partners of these high risk individuals are at risk, as well as any children born to women who carry the virus. Heterosexual persons are increasingly at risk.

AIDS: What Is Safe

MOST BEHAVIOR IS SAFE

Everyday living does not present any risk of infection. You *cannot* get AIDS from casual social contact. Casual social contact should not be confused with casual *sexual* contact which is a major cause of the spread of the AIDS virus. Casual *social* contact such as shaking hands, hugging, social kissing, crying, coughing or sneezing, will not transmit the AIDS virus. Nor has AIDS been contracted from swimming in pools or bathing in hot tubs or from eating in restaurants (even if a restaurant worker has AIDS or carries the AIDS virus). AIDS is not contracted from sharing bed linens, towels, cups, straws, dishes, or any other eating utensils. You cannot get AIDS from toilets, doorknobs, telephones, office machinery, or household furniture. You cannot get AIDS from body massages, masturbation or any non-sexual contact.

DONATING BLOOD

Donating blood is *not* risky at all. *You cannot get AIDS by donating blood.*

RECEIVING BLOOD

In the U.S. every blood donor is screened to exclude high risk persons and every blood donation is now tested for the presence of antibodies to the AIDS virus. Blood that shows exposure to the AIDS virus by the presence of antibodies is not used either for transfusion or for the manufacture of blood products. Blood banks are as safe as current technology can make them. Because antibodies do not form immediately after exposure to the virus, a newly infected person may unknowingly donate blood after becoming infected but before his/her antibody test becomes positive. It is estimated that this might occur less than once in 100,000 donations.

There is no danger of AIDS virus infection from visiting a doctor, dentist, hospital, hairdresser or beautician. AIDS cannot be transmitted non-sexually from an infected person through a health or service provider to another person. Ordinary methods of disinfection for urine, stool and vomitus which are used for non-infected people are adequate for people who have AIDS or are carrying the AIDS virus. You may have wondered why your dentist wears gloves and perhaps a mask when treating you. This does not mean that he has AIDS or that he thinks you do. He is protecting you and himself from hepatitis, common colds or flu.

There is no danger in visiting a patient with AIDS or caring for him or her. Normal hygienic practices, like wiping of body fluid spills with a solution of water and household bleach (1 part household bleach to 10 parts water), will provide full protection.

CHILDREN IN SCHOOL

None of the identified cases of AIDS in the United States are known or are suspected to have been transmitted from one child to another in school, day care, or foster care settings. Transmission would necessitate exposure of open cuts to the blood or other body fluids of the infected child, a highly unlikely occurrence. Even then routine safety procedures for handling blood or other body fluids (which should be standard for all children in the school or day care setting) would be effective in preventing transmission from children with AIDS to other children in school.

Children with AIDS are highly susceptible to infections, such as chicken pox, from other children. Each child with AIDS should be examined by a doctor before attending school or before returning to school, day care or foster care settings after an illness. No blanket rules can be made for all school boards to cover all possible cases of children with AIDS and each case should be considered separately and individualized to the child and the setting, as would be done with any child with a special problem, such as cerebral palsy or asthma. A good team to make such decisions with the school board would be the child's parents, physician and a public health official.

Casual social contact between children and persons infected with the AIDS virus is not dangerous.

INSECTS

There are no known cases of AIDS transmission by insects, such as mosquitoes.

PETS

Dogs, cats and domestic animals are not a source of infection from AIDS virus.

TEARS AND SALIVA

Although the AIDS virus has been found in tears and saliva, no instance of transmission from these body fluids has been reported.

AIDS comes from sexual contacts with infected persons and from the sharing of syringes and needles. There is no danger of infection with AIDS virus by casual social contact.

TESTING OF MILITARY PERSONNEL

You may wonder why the Department of Defense is currently testing its uniformed services personnel for presence of the AIDS virus antibody. The military feel this procedure is necessary because the uniformed services act as their own blood bank in a time of national emergency. They also need to protect new recruits (who unknowingly may be AIDS virus carriers) from receiving live virus vaccines. These vaccines could activate disease and be potentially life-threatening to the recruits.

AIDS: What Is Currently Understood

Although AIDS is still a mysterious disease in many ways, our scientists have learned a great deal about it. In five years we know more about AIDS than many diseases that we have studied for even longer periods. While there is no vaccine or cure, the results from the health and behavioral research community can only add to our knowledge and increase our understanding of the disease and ways to prevent and treat it.

In spite of all that is known about transmission of the AIDS virus, scientists will learn more. One possibility is the potential discovery of factors that may better explain the mechanism of AIDS infection.

Why are the antibodies produced by the body to fight the AIDS virus not able to destroy that virus?

The antibodies detected in the blood of carriers of the AIDS virus are ineffective, at least when classic AIDS is actually triggered. They cannot check the damage caused by the virus, which is by then present in large numbers in the body. Researchers cannot explain this important observation. We still do not know why the AIDS virus is not destroyed by man's immune system.

Summary

AIDS no longer is the concern of any one segment of society; it is the concern of us all. No American's life is in danger if he/she or their sexual partners do not engage in high risk sexual behavior or use shared needles or syringes to inject illicit drugs into the body.

People who engage in high risk sexual behavior or who shoot drugs are risking infection with the AIDS virus and are risking their lives and the lives of others, including their unborn children.

We cannot yet know the full impact of AIDS on our society. From a clinical point of view, there may be new manifestations of AIDS—for example, mental disturbances due to the infection of the brain by the AIDS virus in carriers of the virus. From a social point of view, it may bring to an end the free-wheeling sexual lifestyle which has been called the sexual revolution. Economically, the care of AIDS patients will put a tremendous strain on our already overburdened and costly health care delivery system.

The most certain way to avoid getting the AIDS virus and to control the AIDS epidemic in the United States is for individuals to avoid promiscuous sexual practices, to maintain mutually faithful monogamous sexual relationships and to avoid injecting illicit drugs.

Look to the Future

THE CHALLENGE OF THE FUTURE

An enormous challenge to public health lies ahead of us and we would do well to take a look at the future. We must be prepared to manage those things we can predict, as well as those we cannot.

At the present time there is no vaccine to prevent AIDS. There is no cure. AIDS, which can be transmitted sexually and by sharing needles and syringes among illicit intravenous drug users, is bound to produce profound changes in our society, changes that will affect us all.

INFORMATION AND EDUCATION ONLY WEAPONS AGAINST AIDS

It is estimated that in 1991 54,000 people will die from AIDS. At this moment, many of them are not infected with the AIDS virus. With proper information and education, as many as 12,000 to 14,000 people could be saved in 1991 from death by AIDS.

AIDS WILL IMPACT ALL

The changes in our society will be economic and political and will affect our social institutions, our educational practices, and our health care. Although AIDS may never touch you personally, the societal impact certainly will.

BE EDUCATED—BE PREPARED

Be prepared. Learn as much about AIDS as you can. Learn to separate scientific information from rumor and myth. The Public Health Service, your local public health officials and your family physician will be able to help you.

CONCERN ABOUT SPREAD OF AIDS

While the concentration of AIDS cases is in the larger urban areas today, it has been found in every state and with the mobility of our society, it is likely that cases of AIDS will appear far and wide.

Special Educational Concerns

There are a number of people, primarily adolescents, that do not yet know they will be homosexual or become drug abusers and will not heed this message; there are others who are illiterate and cannot heed this message. They must be reached and taught the risk behaviors that expose them to infection with the AIDS virus.

High Risk Get Blood Test

The greatest public health problem lies in the large number of individuals with a history of high risk behavior who have been infected with and may be spreading the AIDS virus. Those with high risk behavior must be encouraged to protect others by adopting safe sexual practices and by the use of clean equipment for intravenous drug use. If a blood test for antibodies to the AIDS virus is necessary to get these individuals to use safe sexual practices, they should get a blood test. Call your local health department for information on where to get the test.

Anger and Guilt

Some people afflicted with AIDS will feel a sense of anger and others a sense of guilt. In spite of these understandable reactions, everyone must join the effort to control the epidemic, to provide for the care of those with AIDS, and to do all we can to inform and educate others about AIDS, and how to prevent it.

Confidentiality

Because of the stigma that has been associated with AIDS, many afflicted with the disease or who are infected with the AIDS virus are reluctant to be identified with AIDS. Because there is no vaccine to prevent AIDS and no cure, many feel there is nothing to be gained by revealing sexual contacts that might also be infected with the AIDS virus. When a community or a state requires reporting of those infected with the AIDS virus to public health authorities in order to trace sexual and intravenous drug contacts—as is the practice with other sexually transmitted diseases—those infected with the AIDS virus go underground out of the mainstream of health care and education. For this reason current public health practice is to protect the privacy of the individual infected with the AIDS virus and to maintain the strictest confidentiality concerning his/her health records.

STATE AND LOCAL AIDS TASK FORCES

Many state and local jurisdictions where AIDS has been seen in the greatest numbers have AIDS task forces with heavy representation from the field of public health joined by others who can speak broadly to issues of access to care, provision of care and the availability of community and psychiatric support services. Such a task force is needed in every community with the power to develop plans and policies, to speak, and to act for the good of the public health at every level.

State and local task forces should plan ahead and work collaboratively with other jurisdictions to reduce transmission of AIDS by far-reaching informational and educational programs. As AIDS impacts more strongly on society, they should be charged with making recommendations to provide for the needs of those afflicted with AIDS. They also will be in the best position to answer the concerns and direct the activities of those who are not infected with the AIDS virus.

The responsibility of state and local task forces should be far reaching and might include the following areas:
• Insure enforcement of public health regulation of such practices as ear piercing and tattooing to prevent transmission of the AIDS virus.
• Conduct AIDS education programs for police, firemen, correctional institution workers and emergency medical personnel for dealing with AIDS victims and the public.
• Insure that institutions catering to children or adults who soil themselves or their surroundings with urine, stool, and vomitus have adequate equipment for cleanup and disposal, and have policies to insure the practice of good hygiene.

SCHOOL

Schools will have special problems in the future. In addition to the guidelines already mentioned in this pamphlet, there are other things that should be considered such as sex education and education of the handicapped.

Sex Education

Education concerning AIDS must start at the lowest grade possible as part of any health and hygiene program. The appearance of AIDS could bring together diverse groups of parents and educators with opposing views on inclusion of sex education in the curricula. There is now no doubt that we need sex education in schools and that it must include information on heterosexual and homosexual relationships. The threat of AIDS should be sufficient to permit a sex education curriculum with a heavy emphasis on prevention of AIDS and other sexually transmitted diseases.

Handicapped and Special Education

Children with AIDS or ARC will be attending school along with others who carry the AIDS virus. Some children will develop brain disease which will produce changes in mental behavior. Because of the right to special education of the handicapped and the mentally retarded, school boards and higher authorities will have to provide guidelines for the management of such children on a case-by-case basis.

Labor and Management

Labor and management can do much to prepare for AIDS so that misinformation is kept to a minimum. Unions should issue preventive health messages because many employees will listen more carefully to a union message than they will to one from public health authorities.

AIDS Education at the Work Site

Offices, factories, and other work sites should have a plan in operation for education of the work force and accommodation of AIDS or ARC patients *before* the first such case appears at the work site. Employees with AIDS or ARC should be dealt with as are any workers with a chronic illness. In-house video programs provide an excellent source of education and can be individualized to the needs of a specific work group.

STRAIN ON THE HEALTH CARE DELIVERY SYSTEM

The health care system in many places will be overburdened as it is now in urban areas with large numbers of AIDS patients. It is predicted that during 1991 there will be 145,000 patients requiring hospitalization at least once and 54,000 patients who will die of AIDS. Mental disease (dementia) will occur in some patients who have the AIDS virus before they have any other manifestation such as ARC or classic AIDS.

State and local task forces will have to plan for these patients by utilizing conventional and time honored systems but will also have to investigate alternate methods of treatment and alternate sites for care including homecare.

The strain on the health system can be lessened by family, social, and psychological support mechanisms in the community. Programs are needed to train chaplains, clergy, social workers, and volunteers to deal with AIDS. Such support is particularly critical to the minority communities.

MENTAL HEALTH

Our society will also face an additional burden as we better understand the mental health implications of infection by the AIDS virus. Upon being informed of infection with the AIDS virus, a young, active, vigorous person faces anxiety and depression brought on by fears associated with social isolation, illness, and dying. Dealing with these individual and family concerns will require the best efforts of mental health professionals.

CONTROVERSIAL ISSUES

A number of controversial AIDS issues have arisen and will continue to be debated largely because of lack of knowledge about AIDS, how it is spread, and how it can be prevented. Among these are the issues of compulsory blood testing, quarantine, and identification of AIDS carriers by some visible sign.

COMPULSORY BLOOD TESTING

Compulsory blood testing of individuals is not necessary. The procedure could be unmanageable and cost prohibitive. It can be expected that many who *test* negatively might actually be positive due to *recent* exposure to the AIDS virus and give a false sense of security to the individual and his/her sexual partners concerning necessary protective behavior. The prevention behavior described in this report, if adopted, will protect the American public and contain the AIDS epidemic. Voluntary testing will be available to those who have been involved in high risk behavior.

Quarantine

Quarantine has no role in the management of AIDS because AIDS is not spread by casual contact. The only time that some form of quarantine might be indicated is in a situation where an individual carrying the AIDS virus knowingly and willingly continues to expose others through sexual contact or sharing drug equipment. Such circumstances should be managed on a case-by-case basis by local authorities.

Identification of AIDS Carriers by Some Visible Sign

Those who suggest the marking of carriers of the AIDS virus by some visible sign have not thought the matter through thoroughly. It would require testing of the entire population which is unnecessary, unmanageable and costly. It would miss those recently infected individuals who would test negatively, but be infected. The entire procedure would give a false sense of security. AIDS must and will be treated as a disease that can infect anyone. AIDS should not be used as an excuse to discriminate against any group or individual.

Updating Information

As the Surgeon General, I will continually monitor the most current and accurate health, medical, and scientific information and make it available to you, the American people. Armed with this information you can join in the discussion and resolution of AIDS-related issues that are critical to your health, your children's health, and the health of the nation.

Additional Information

TELEPHONE HOTLINES (TOLL FREE)

PHS AIDS Hotline: 800-342-AIDS, 800-342-2437

National Sexually Transmitted Diseases Hotline/American Social Health Association: 800-227-8922

National Gay Task Force, AIDS Information Hotline: 800-221-7044, (212) 807-6016 (NY State)

INFORMATION SOURCES

U.S. Public Health Service Public Affairs Office, Hubert H. Humphrey Building, Room 725-H, 200 Independence Avenue, S.W., Washington, D.C. 20201. Phone: (202) 245-6867

Local Red Cross or American Red Cross AIDS Education Office, 1730 D Street, N.W., Washington, D.C. 20006. Phone: (202) 737-8300

American Association of Physicians for Human Rights, P.O. Box 14366, San Francisco, CA 94114. Phone: (415) 558-9353

AIDS Action Council, 729 Eighth Street, S.E., Suite 200, Washington, D.C. 20003. Phone: (202) 547-3101

Gay Men's Health Crisis, P.O. Box 274, 132 West 24th Street, New York, NY 10011. Phone: (212) 807-6655

Hispanic AIDS Forum, c/o APRED, 853 Broadway, Suite 2007, New York, NY 10003. Phone: (212) 870-1902 or 870-1864

Los Angeles AIDS Project, 1362 Santa Monica Boulevard, Los Angeles, California, 90046. (213) 871-AIDS

Minority Task Force on AIDS, c/o New York City Council of Churches, 475 Riverside Drive, Room 456, New York, NY 10115. Phone: (212) 749-1214

Mothers of AIDS Patients (MAP), c/o Barbara Peabody, 3403 E Street, San Diego, CA 92102. Phone: (619) 234-3432

National AIDS Network, 729 Eighth Street, S.E., Suite 300, Washington, D.C. 20003. Phone: (202) 546-2424

National Association of People with AIDS, P.O. Box 65472, Washington, D.C. 20035. Phone: (202) 483-7979

National Coalition of Gay Sexually Transmitted Disease Services, c/o Mark Behar, P.O. Box 239, Milwaukee, WI 53201. Phone: (414) 277-7671

National Council of Churches/AIDS Task Force, 475 Riverside Drive, Room 572, New York, NY 10115. Phone: (212) 870-2421

San Francisco AIDS Foundation, 333 Valencia Street, 4th Floor, San Francisco, CA 94103. Phone: (415) 863-2437

II. AIDS VICTIMS AND RESEARCH

EDITOR'S INTRODUCTION

For the thousands of AIDS victims, those at risk, and their friends and families, anxiety over the AIDS epidemic has been intense. How are those directly affected to cope, and how can medical personnel deal, with the AIDS crisis? What treatment and drugs are now being developed that may offer hope of containing the progress of the disease? Section II examines these issues in a series of articles by journalists and professionals in the health care field.

Glen Allen's article from *Maclean's* focuses on the devastating effect of AIDS on gays in Canadian cities, while noting how the announcement by Rock Hudson of his having AIDS has spurred interest in the AIDS crisis. In *American Psychologist,* Anthony J. Ferrara relates his personal ordeal, an article made poignant by the editor's announcement at the end of Ferrara's death. Another article by medical professionals Stephen F. Morin and Walter F. Batchelor, in the journal *Public Health Reports,* published by the U. S. Public Health Service, deals with the severe psychological problems that accompany the "mysterious and stigmatized illness," and that require the attention of mental health staffs and community volunteers.

The latter part of this section looks at the new techniques for fighting AIDS. Two articles, by Pat Ohlendorf in *Maclean's* and Annabel Hecht in the *FDA Consumer,* survey a wide variety of drugs in an experimental stage, but conclude pessimistically that none offers hope of an imminent cure. Scott Ticer's report in *Business Week* reveals the existence of a "black market" of drugs available in Mexico but not in the U.S., and other panaceas on which the desperate are spending millions. Denise Grady, in an article from *Discover,* discusses the most touted of the AIDS drugs, AZT. Although AZT does not cure AIDS, it has been effective in laboratory tests in halting its multiplication, and may soon be released on the market. Finally, Peter Huber, writing in *New Republic,* points out that if a vaccine were to be developed (and none is as yet in view), litigation resulting from its possible side effects might well intimidate any pharmaceutical company from making it available.

THE NEW TERROR OF AIDS[1]

Pierre-Donat Robitaille's birthday party last year began with a joke: 10 of his friends decorated a vanilla cake with 49 candles—11 more than his age. But the joke turned out badly because Robitaille, a bartender in downtown Toronto, was hardly able to blow the candles out. And two days later he was admitted to Toronto's Mount Sinai Hospital with a rare form of pneumonia. Then, doctors told him the devastating news: he had contracted acquired immune deficiency syndrome (AIDS), the incurable condition that has already claimed 145 lives in Canada during the past three years and is assuming epidemic proportions around the world. Now, with screen idol Rock Hudson stricken by the usually fatal disease, AIDS has finally become an openly discussed, potentially terrifying international preoccupation.

Miracle: For his part, Robitaille this week faces another birthday, almost alone and knowing that it will likely be his last. He has a gaunt appearance, his face has a grey pallor and he has had to struggle constantly against depression. Said Robitaille: "I have lost 80 per cent of my friends." Indeed, AIDS has stripped Robitaille of nearly everything he holds dear. He has lost his job (his employer told him that his condition was "not good for business") and his lover left him, Robitaille said, "because he did not want to die." And last week, surrounded by the stained-glass windows he makes as a hobby, Robitaille said he would hope for a miracle on his birthday. He added, "I will wish for a cure for AIDS—if not for me, then for those who will get it soon."

Robitaille has been reduced to living on welfare payments of $375 per month, afflicted by a disease that has spread with devastating swiftness through homosexual communities since U.S. researchers identified the condition four years ago. At the same time, fear and concern over AIDS has risen as the number of vic-

[1]Reprint of an article by Glen Allen. *Maclean's*. Reprinted by permission from *Maclean's*, 98:35. Ag. 12, '85. Copyright © 1985 by *Maclean's*.

tims increased, as researchers discovered that heterosexuals could catch the disease through sexual contact—or even from a victim's saliva—and as AIDS carriers transmitted the condition to new victims through blood transfusions. Then, late last month the disease acquired a new visibility as Hudson, the Hollywood film star of the 1950s and 1960s, and more recently a TV star as well, announced in Paris that he had AIDS.

Hudson had travelled to France in the hope that an antiviral substance being tested at the Pasteur Clinic would cure his condition. Then, last week he flew back to California aboard an Air France 747 jet chartered at a cost of $250,000. But his haggard appearance on television news reports and in newspaper photographs of the former leading man produced a wave of sympathy for all AIDS victims and created a surge of interest in the search for a cure. To that end, several of Hudson's friends in Hollywood, among them Elizabeth Taylor, Burt Lancaster and Burt Reynolds, announced that they were planning a benefit performance next month with the goal of raising $1 million to combat AIDS.

As he tried to regain his dwindling strength in a Los Angeles clinic—with a get-well card from U.S. President Ronald Reagan nearby—Hudson's condition had clearly accomplished some good. For one thing, the announcement linked a famous face and name to AIDS' grim and lengthening columns of statistics. In the United States more than 12,000 victims have contracted the disease which almost invariably kills them within three years. In New York state alone, where almost 4,000 cases have been reported, AIDS has become the leading cause of death for men between 25 and 44. Declared Richard Dunne, executive director of the Gay Men's Health Crisis, a counselling and health service for homosexuals: "I know 20 to 30 people who have died. I do not know if my mother knows as many friends or acquaintances who have died."

Suspect: The numbers are much smaller in Canada, where doctors have diagnosed 288 cases of AIDS during the past three years. Of those, 145 have already proved fatal. And Dr. Alastair Clayton of the federal Laboratory Centre for Disease Control in Ottawa estimated that doctors had not reported as many as 90 cases of the disease. Indeed, federal health officials suspect that as many as 24,000 Canadians may be carriers of AIDS antibodies. There are now an estimated one million carriers of AIDS antibodies in North America alone, prompting Dr. Robert Redfield, a researcher at the Walter Reed Institute in Washington, D.C., to declare: "This is a general disease now. Anyone could catch it."

In Hudson's case, he began experiencing the early symptoms of AIDS, fatigue and weight loss, nearly two years ago. Doctors soon discovered that he had, at least, a form of the disease, but they allowed him to honor his commitment to appear in six episodes of the *Dynasty* television series. Last month when he flew to Paris he did not initially tell even the doctors at the American Hospital that he had AIDS. That, in turn, led to confused reports about his condition until Hudson himself made the decision to announce the nature of his illness publicly.

Surgery: Hudson's homosexuality had been a closely guarded Hollywood secret which, if it had become known, would have destroyed the macho image that he developed in scores of movies, such as *Magnificent Obsession* in 1954. But friends say he frequently visited gay bars and went on occasional drinking sprees.

If sexual promiscuity and carelessness were seen during the days of "gay liberation" as the hallmarks of North America's homosexual communities, the spectre of AIDS has given them a sober sense of co-operation and even collective bravery nowhere more than in San Francisco, where the disease is a political, as well as a public health issue. There, 667 of 1,307 AIDS victims have died so far in a city where an estimated 70,000 homosexuals form one of the largest and most influential communities in North America.

Fear of contracting AIDS has affected bathhouses and clubs which thrived by offering places for casual sex. Now a steep drop in business has forced 12 baths and sex clubs to close down, and those remaining have abandoned such practices as providing "glory holes" for anonymous sexual encounters. Instead, club owners are now urging their customers to use condoms during intercourse—or suggesting that they indulge in mutual masturbation, a practice that does not carry the risk of contracting AIDS through the exchange of semen or saliva.

'Victims': At the same time, San Francisco health officials have noted a decline in the number of cases of other sexually transmitted diseases such as gonorrhea—in part, they say, because many homosexuals have stopped performing anal intercourse. And in a June telephone survey which polled 500 homosexual and bisexual men, the city's AIDS Foundation found

that eight out of 10 respondents said they had made dramatic
changes in their sexual behavior and now stressed safe sex practices. Said Randy Shilts, a reporter who regularly writes about
AIDS for *The San Francisco Chronicle*: "Being sleazy is just passé.
It is a whole different ball game now. The biggest gay gatherings
are at Alcoholics Anonymous, with people trying to get off the
fast track. And many gay men have become involved in counselling groups and volunteer work to help AIDS victims."

Fear: The preference for safer sex is also growing in Vancouver's homosexual community. In Neighbor's, a well-appointed
nightclub heavily patronized by homosexuals, assistant manager
William Harvey estimated that the club's revenue has dropped by
30 per cent during the past year. Still, his club remains open, unlike two nearby steambaths in the crowded West End of the city
which closed because of poor business. Harvey cited AIDS as the
cause. He added: "We had five customers die of it last year. There
is a lot less cruising now—people are taking more time to get to
know each other. Before, you could go home on a handshake."

Customers sitting on the other side of the bar confirmed Harvey's observations. Said a 30-year-old office employee with the
federal government: "AIDS has affected my life very deeply—
and the way I look at people and relationships. Two of my friends
have it." Others agreed, stressing that fear of contracting the disease has led them to change their sexual practices. Added Bruce
Smyth, the co-owner of Little Sisters, a West End bookstore
which caters to homosexuals: "I certainly do not have anal sex
anymore without a safe [condom]. And I have cut down on the
number of my sexual partners."

There have been similar discussions in bars, restaurants, clubs
and living rooms throughout the continent. And following Hudson's disclosure and the remarkable wave of sympathy it produced, AIDS victims came forward to tell their story. Among
them:

• Walter lives in Montreal and, fearing recognition, declined to
give his full name. When he spoke at an AIDS conference at the
University of Quebec last May he cloaked himself in a white hospital gown and black goggles. He has lived with AIDS for two
years and he has suffered through several associated diseases, including pneumonia, and now cancer. Like many other sufferers,
he is not only very sick but broke and isolated as well. And last
week he described his life with a degree of bitterness. Said Wal-

ter: "What I can say is that last week I had AIDS. This week I have Rock Hudson's disease. I wish he had publicly come out with it a year ago, because maybe a lot more funding and interest and communications would have happened. But at least it is happening now."

Walter lives on a disability insurance payment of $440 a month, which he says is "far from fair." When he learned that he had AIDS he said he was "totally devastated by the death sentence it implied, by the physical pain and discomfort and by the isolation." He added, "I had a lot of hard times in the hospital because the staff was afraid to come into my room." And he had more trouble still finding a dentist who would treat his decaying teeth. Indeed, no dentist would approach him "and now my teeth are totally destroyed. The decay has gone right to the bone."

Still, Walter said that he found comfort in the company of others with AIDS. He added: "The first two people I met who had it are now dead. But I recently met some other people who look like they are going to be around for a bit. The anguish—the emotional anguish, the mental anguish and of course the physical. AIDS means death."

• Allan Pletcher, a Vancouver community college teacher, learned that he had AIDS three months ago. He already suspected that his body carried the virus, and for four years he was tired and wracked by a bad cough that still convulses his body. When doctors at Vancouver's St. Paul's Hospital told him last May that he had only about a year to live he said that "I took it as death sentence." Since then, he said, he has learned to accept and to fight his condition, encouraged by stories of sufferers who have lived as many as four years after their diagnosis. But the scene of his inevitable deathbed still haunts his imagination. He wants to die in his own Victorian bed, under his handcrafted quilt and surrounded by friends. Added Pletcher: "I am concerned that I will be in pain or in a coma. I want to die in my own room and be conscious. I fear dying but not death."

More fortunate than most AIDS sufferers, Pletcher lives on a $480 weekly disability payment and sometimes he is able to dine out with friends. Still, one recent dinner host asked him if he would mind eating off a paper plate. Said Pletcher: "I was hurt, but I understand the fear that is around."

• James Black, 37, of Toronto said that he believes he caught the lethal virus last August after he had anal intercourse with a South

African whom he met through an advertisement placed in *The Toronto Star*. In September he collapsed with exhaustion and physicians at Toronto's Wellesley Hospital told him that he had either malaria or AIDS. It was not until January, after more bouts of illness, that Dr. Jenny Heathcote of Toronto Western Hospital told Black, "It's AIDS." Black asked, "Is it buy-the-casket and order-the-flowers time?" The answer, although unstated, was yes. He is expected to die this fall.

Black has dropped to 120 lb. from his former weight of 186 and has brain seizures, bronchitis and yeast infections on his hands and mouth. But his spirit lives in the T-shirt he wears, which boldly proclaims "Choose Life." Said Black: "Don't feel sorry for me. I know what I have and I have accepted it. I am not ashamed—unlucky, yes, but not ashamed." Many of Black's friends have deserted him, and when he applied for a disability pension a Toronto welfare worker told him, "You may not live long enough to make the paperwork worthwhile." Black is giving whatever energy he can manage to his duty as a spokesman for the AIDS Committee of Toronto.

One friend who has not deserted Black is his roommate, 19-year-old Kevin Stacey, a Toronto department store clerk. In caring for Black, Stacey carefully scalds their dishware. Indeed, he has few illusions about the risks that he faces. Said Stacey: "It is scary but I am well informed, and that is the message I want to get across to people. I asked myself, 'Should I take off or should I handle this with the dignity he deserves?' It was the least I could do. I love him so much."

• AIDS sufferer Edward McLaren, 31, a former University of British Columbia student of landscape architecture, faces his fate with composure. Said McLaren: "Life isn't really all that different when you have a disease like this. You either carry on and get as much out of it as you can or you curl up in a corner and cry the blues." But for McLaren, carrying on means living with neurological distress—including memory loss and loss of balance—headaches and a dramatically reduced lung capacity because of a bout with pneumocystis pneumonia, a common AIDS complication. His doctor told him last September that he had AIDS but the news did not surprise him. Said McLaren: "My sinuses had been giving me problems all summer. I had gone for my regular checkup and the balance of cells was way out. A good sign of AIDS."

McLaren lives on a provincial government handicap pension of $560 a month, supplemented by a monthly Canada Pension payment of $250. But his life is made more bearable by the continuing support of family and friends. Several friends visit regularly to talk "about the deep, dark mystery of AIDS." And when he was released from an eight-week stay in hospital last fall six friends took turns cooking his supper each night.

Struck: For every AIDS sufferer still alive and able to tell of his experience, there remains the memory of another victim whom the disease has silenced forever. Within the Erickson family of Fort St. John, a small community in northern British Columbia, that memory is still fresh. Louise Ann Erickson was in the prime of life when she died two weeks ago at 40, leaving behind a husband and two preteen children. She remained healthy until a month before her death, but she was struck down suddenly by pneumocystis pneumonia, a consequence of the AIDS virus that had lodged in her body three years ago, probably following blood transfusions during a cancer operation. Three hundred mourners attended a memorial service for Erickson at St. Luke's United Church, and they gave donations for AIDS research that "filled a grocery bag," according to Rev. Ann Foster.

The gesture moved the entire province. Said Foster: "We are trying to take a senseless tragedy and make it a little less senseless." It is a tragedy that is repeating itself with a distressing and increasing frequency at a time when medical practice was never more promising—or more powerless.

MY PERSONAL EXPERIENCE WITH AIDS[2]

Last March, I was diagnosed as having AIDS. This altered my life so profoundly that seven months later I am still struggling to adjust to the change.

[2]Reprint of an article by Anthony J. Ferrara, AIDS victim, *American Psychologist*. Reprinted by permission from *American Psychologist*, pp. 1285–86. N. '84. Copyright © 1984 by *American Psychologist*. This article is drawn from a speech delivered to the National AIDS Forum sponsored by the AIDS Education Fund of the Whitman-Walker Clinic, Washington, DC, on October 8, 1983. Requests for reprints should be sent to Walter F. Batchelor, Program Officer for Health Policy. American Psychological Association, 1200 Seventeenth Street, N.W., Washington, D.C. 20036.

Perhaps my reaction was different from most AIDS patients. Because we are all individuals, I am sure that every person so diagnosed reacts differently. No one can fully understand another's anguish in such circumstances; no one can fully comprehend the pain. Nevertheless, let me recount my personal experience, although cautioning against accepting it as "normal" for all other AIDS patients.

Suspecting that the purple spots that appeared on the inside of my thighs might be Kaposi's sarcoma, I tried to prepare myself for the news that would be given by my doctor. I asked to be informed of the results of the biopsy as soon as possible, even if it had to be given to me over the phone. As it turned out, that was the way I received my diagnosis.

The doctor was very compassionate, saying that this was probably the worst news I had ever received in my life, and he was right. All of my mental preparation was insufficient to thwart the tidal wave of emotion that swept over me as I received what, at the time, I regarded as a death sentence. I went home that evening in the company of my lover Michael, feeling the weight of two worlds—mine and his—on my shoulders.

Wanting to protect him not only from the possibility of contracting the disease himself, but also from the difficulties that I knew were ahead for me, I asked him to leave me. He refused, reminding me that we were in this together.

Initially, Michael took the news worse than I. As I look back on those days now, I realize that I didn't have time to think of myself; I was too busy taking care of him. But as time went on, things began to work their way back into perspective.

I have always considered myself an independent person, tough enough to brave everything life had to throw at me. In fact, I took pride in my ability to "tough things out"—alone, if necessary. And that was the way I wanted it. "To fade into the sunset," I believe is the way I expressed it to Michael. Because he wasn't about to leave me and was not, as he said, "strong enough to go it alone," we decided to confide in a small circle of friends for support.

Michael cried, I guess, for about six weeks—to the point that my own emotion had to be contained. Actually, because of the way in which he was dealing with the problem, I *was* going it alone. Eventually we were able to cry together, although I still feel ashamed and weak at such emotional displays. It is OK, from my perspective, for other people to cry, but not for me. It has not been easy allowing myself the relief—the freedom—such crying brings.

The Whitman-Walker Clinic in Washington has provided counseling services through the St. Francis Center, which I have found very valuable. My counselor is a professional who understands that being depressed is not so bad, but is rather a normal mental experience. She also understands when I am not "up," as so many of my friends, and my lover, expected me to be at their slightest urging.

It is also extremely difficult for me to make others understand that I do not want sympathy. It is demeaning and humiliating to me when I perceive that someone feels sorry for me. Friends can be supportive, understanding and helpful without pitying me.

For the most part, my friends continue to be supportive. There also seems to have developed a group of new acquaintances offering to do whatever they can to help in my new and unfortunate circumstances. Some friends have grown in other directions, but mostly because of the dynamics of their own lives, rather than because of any reluctance to associate with a friend who has AIDS. But, as my energies have waned and my hospitalizations have curtailed my availability for social encounters, our lives seem to have grown apart. My feelings about this are mixed. On the one hand, as my illness progresses, my need for emotional support increases: on the other, I dislike the feeling that my friends are pitying me.

For those of you with friends with AIDS, please remember that this is no time for an "out of sight, out of mind" philosophy. When your friends are too ill to participate in your life as they did before, don't just forget them. Remember, this is when they need you the most and, if you can, respond to that need.

Probably the most heartbreaking thing for me has been the realization that physical fitness and other abilities I have always taken for granted are becoming more difficult to maintain, and my daily regimen has become more and more of an effort.

Four months prior to my diagnosis, I ran the Marine Corps Marathon in about 4 hours. At the time of my diagnosis, I was running between 4 and 12 miles a day, working out on weights 3 times a week, and attending aerobics class almost every day. Additionally, I maintained a natural, almost entirely vegetarian diet and took lots of vitamins. Obviously, maintaining your health is not an adequate precaution against contracting AIDS.

Struggling to maintain my physical conditioning through all the emotional and physical realities, plus the debilitating treatments, has called upon all of my resources. It is difficult for me to run even two miles now, although I continue to do so. Weight training is still reasonably easy for me, and walking is good also. When I am on intravenous medication, I try to ride a stationary bicycle that has been placed in my room at the hospital.

All of this is possible. However, it is sometimes very difficult to muster the motivation to do this when I am weak and depressed.

After my diagnosis, I was referred to the National Institutes of Health for study and treatment. Since then, I have been in and out of the hospital on a regular basis, the latest hospital stint lasting two months.

The doctors, nurses, and support staff at NIH are extremely compassionate, dedicated, and professional. There really is no way I can adequately express my gratitude for these people and their efforts to save the lives of the AIDS patients there. Researchers first and foremost, they nevertheless make every effort to address the myriad problems we face in coping with a life-threatening illness, including counseling, answering just about any question put to them, and patiently enduring our anger when our own anxieties get the better of us. They are, in the final analysis, genuine humanitarians, facing all the frustrations incorporated in researching an unknown and baffling killer that is so complex that leads toward a possible cure or treatment dissolve as quickly as they appear.

That is, I guess, the greatest frustration—knowing that there is virtually nothing we can do or say that will change the situation much. I have been a part of four different protocols, or experimental treatments, and have shown improvement on three of them. However, my progress was not sufficient to warrant continuation of any of them.

The first began in late April—treatments with Alpha Interferon. The protocol required 10 daily injections, 10 days of rest, and then 10 more daily injections. The side effects were both physically and emotionally devastating. Within two hours of the first injection, I had severe chills, followed by high fever, and reversion back to chills. The evening of the first injection, my fever climbed to 104 degrees, and there were a few hours when I scarcely remember anything.

These side effects subsided after a few days, but the most devastating side effects were still to come. Over the 30-day course of treatment, aside from a brief respite during the 10-day rest period, I noticed myself becoming profoundly more fatigued and depressed. Just before the course of interferon treatment I was still running 4 miles a day; now there were days that I barely wanted to get out of bed.

It was at this point that I finally realized what was going to happen to me—I was going to die. From the first moment of that realization to this very day, it is not the act of passing from life to death that frightens me but the events that lead up to that point. The body and physical abilities of which I have been so proud and for which I have worked so hard are deteriorating with cancer and weakness.

The next treatment was with Gamma Interferon, another of the interferons made from a different type of blood cell. Gamma Interferon involved 28 days of a daily two-hour intravenous infusion. There were few side effects, but there was also no progress. During this period the number of cancer lesions on my body increased dramatically. The interferon itself did not cause weakness, but my level of fitness and personal well-being continued to decline.

Over the last two months, beginning August 1, I have had 13 total plasma exchanges—a process called plasmapheresis—and a 28-day cycle of Interleukin II.

Plasma exchange is a very taxing procedure, involving the removal of almost all the blood in the body over a 5-hour period, spinning it, removing the old plasma, mixing the remaining blood cells with new plasma, and returning it to the body. With plasma exchange, there is the chance that the patient will react to certain properties in the new plasma. This happened to me during my fourth plasma exchange. The reaction consisted of violent chills—so severe that my body was actually involuntarily jumping off the bed. My physician was with me at the time, and all I really remember about the experience was looking up at him and asking if I was going to die. He assured me that I wasn't, and I came through it all right.

After the multiple plasma exchanges, I received Interleukin II. It is administered by intravenous injection, 24 hours a day, five days a week for four weeks. The side effects were minimal, but the tube necessary for the continuous intravenous injection restricted movement and, therefore, exercise. My overall fitness, again, deteriorated.

I now have about one month with no treatment planned. I am using this time to try to build my body strength back up—if not to where it was before my treatment began, at least to as close as that state of fitness as possible.

I am convinced that to give up is to die. For this reason I submit my body and my life to further experimentation because there simply isn't anything else to do. It is only a matter of time until this research renders answers, treatments, and cures. For those of us already afflicted, it is a matter of holding on until research efforts are successful. That is our hope. Although there are discouraging moments, we cannot—we will not—lose sight of that hope.

To those of you not afflicted goes the task of ensuring that our cause is not forgotten by the politicians and civic leaders responsible for allocating funds to carry on the research that feeds our hopes. To you is assigned the work of keeping our plight in the public eye so that those who would ignore the problem in the hope that it will go away, or those who would declare it to be a problem afflicting only a single segment of our society, cannot accomplish what people of good conscience know is patently wrong. It is up to you to correct the public's misperception, fostered by often insensitive media representation, that all AIDS patients are ignoble, drug-abusing people who are undeserving of attention, let alone the benefits of a worldwide quest to save them from a devastating disease.

We are not bad people. We are merely gay, and that is no reason to regard us with disdain. Those of us physically unable to carry on this message look to you for champions.

EDITOR'S NOTE: Tony Ferrara died on June 4, 1984.

RESPONDING TO THE PSYCHOLOGICAL CRISIS OF AIDS[3]

Acquired immune deficiency syndrome (AIDS) is most frequently understood as a mysterious and deadly medical phenomenon. It strips a person's immune system of the ability to fight off life-threatening infections and cancers. Now there is a growing awareness that AIDS has profound psychological ramifications as well—with a reach far broader than the disease syndrome itself. These mental health aspects of the AIDS crisis begin with the individual person, expand to friends and family, include health care workers who treat people with AIDS, and have begun to engulf whole segments of society.

First, consider one man's experiences:

For the first time in my life, October 1981, I found myself bedridden with a cold that wouldn't go away, viral bronchitis, fever, diarrhea, loss of appetite, and extreme fatigue. These problems persisted for several months and were coupled with the discovery of swollen lymph nodes, which began to really alarm me. Then I developed chronic ear infections, shingles on the backs of both legs, and a persistent sore throat. The diarrhea continued and nausea became a fact of everyday life; eating became increasingly difficult—I began to lose weight.

I was frightened and depressed by the fact that the illnesses were multiple, and that no sooner would one go away than something else would appear. I then began to experience with increasing frequency the most alarming and intimidating of all these maladies—night sweats. Sometimes I would wake up crying because I was so cold and frightened. No amount of preparation before bed could relieve the anxiety and fear of what was to come. I dreaded what I knew I needed most—sleep; I didn't want to close my eyes.

The initial diagnostic process was probably as confusing and frustrating to the doctors as it was to me. Blood tests and biopsies were always negative or inconclusive; the doctors could only tell me what I didn't have. "Well, it looks like Hodgkin's disease, but it isn't—and it looks like leukemia, but it isn't," etc.

[3]Reprint of an article by Stephen F. Morin, clinical psychologist, and Walter F. Batchelor, program officer for Health Policy, American Psychological Association. Reprinted by permission from *Public Health Reports*, v. 99, 4–9, Ja./F. '84. Copyright © 1984 by U. S. Public Health Service.

They ruled out the likely and even the unlikely possibilities. I still didn't know. Nothing. I had no idea if it was contagious, if it was cureable, if anyone else had it or had ever had it. I was alone, frightened, and confused. I desperately needed help in coping with the emotional turmoil of facing this unknown. Was I going to die?

How should mental health issues related to AIDS be addressed? How can mental health services be integrated into comprehensive health care for people with AIDS? What is the appropriate role for community mental health agencies and alternative self-help approaches? What are the mental health implications of AIDS for lovers, friends, and families of people with AIDS, people with lesser forms of immune suppression, the gay male community in general, and health care providers? We believe that each of these points needs to be discussed.

Since there is little research literature on the psychological aspects of AIDS, we have relied in this paper on our own personal and professional experiences. Most important, we have relied on interviews and written statements from several men who have AIDS, from their lovers, and from other family members. Additionally, we have drawn from the experiences of gay community organizations that are struggling to meet the psychological needs of people with AIDS.

People with AIDS

Eighty-five percent of persons with AIDS are diagnosed with either Kaposi's sarcoma (KS), *Pneumocystis carinii* pneumonia (PCP), or both. These rare conditions were once virtually unheard of outside of medical circles. Now, however, these diagnoses are well-known and generally thought of as being equivalent to a death sentence. The fact that people diagnosed as suffering from AIDS are likely to have major emotional reactions to hearing the diagnosis should be obvious. Apparently, it is not. We have spoken to several men who have received the diagnosis of AIDS over the telephone from their primary care physicians. No attention was paid to the psychological impact of this diagnosis, and no provisions were made to help the man respond to his emotions.

The director of a mental health crisis center told us that the number of AIDS-related calls has increased geometrically over the past 18 months, including an increasing number of calls about threats of suicide or homicide. These calls are from people who have just been diagnosed with AIDS, or from their family members, who do not know what the future will be or if their worst fantasies will come true. The director stressed the need, after crisis intervention, to direct callers to sources of support and to continue to follow these people carefully.

We believe that mental health considerations should be part of all assessment and treatment procedures for people with AIDS. At the point of diagnosis, for instance, the practitioner's awareness of emotional factors can help prevent the patient's natural fear and anger from being transformed into self-destructive expressions. During continuing medical treatment, mental health workers can help develop understanding of the emotional needs of both patient and health professional. Psychological assistance during the stages close to death can bring a depth of caring that supersedes the depression and fear at hand.

The role of mental health care practitioners in the AIDS epidemic must encompass an understanding and willingness to deal with factors that make AIDS different from most other disease states—94 percent of persons with AIDS are also characterized by atypical social labels. Approximately 71 percent are gay or bisexual, 17 percent are users of intravenous drugs, and 5 percent are Haitian. The fact that most persons with AIDS are culturally different from most physicians and mental health professionals places additional burdens on all concerned.

We pay special attention to the largest group affected by AIDS, gay men. If gay men are to receive optimal health care, their primary care physician must be aware of their sexual orientation. A study by Dardick and Grady indicated that 49 percent of the sample population of lesbians and gay men had told their primary health care professional that they were homosexual, and another 11 percent assumed that their practitioner knew. An additional 34 percent would say that they were lesbian or gay if they thought it was important. Only 7 percent would not share this information under any circumstances. Dardick and Grady found that openness led to greater satisfaction with the primary health care providers and that the attitudes of health professionals toward homosexuality were an important concern of the respondents.

The attitude of mental health professionals toward homosexuality is similarly important. Too frequently, psychotherapy has been characterized by a heterosexual bias, that is, a belief that heterosexual orientation is superior to or more natural (or both) than homosexual orientation. This heterosexual bias is reflected in diagnostic assessments, treatment goals, and even the language used in psychotherapy. The fact that some significant percentage of gay men do not feel emotionally supported by their families and may be isolated from other gay men and women makes it imperative that health care professionals look for, identify, and respond to their special psychological needs.

For people with AIDS, psychological needs stem from such psychosocial stressors as fear of death and dying, repeated infections, degenerative physical status, social stigma, fear of exposure of lifestyle, guilt, fear of contagion, loss of lovers or friends, fears of loss of physical attractiveness, loss of occupational and financial status, and increased dependency. Given the number and variety of stressors that may be present and the symptoms that may develop (for example, anxiety, depression, and the cognitive deficits secondary to medical treatment), supportive psychotherapy is generally recommended.

In addition to these psychological problems, being treated as a person with a rare disease and being a participant in medical research can be debilitating. One man with AIDS told us:

My treatment with Alpha Interferon required ten daily injections, ten days of rest and ten more daily injections. Within two hours of the first injection, I had severe chills, followed by high fever, and reversion back to chills. These side effects subsided after a few days, but the most devastating were still to come. Over the 30-day course of treatment, I noticed myself becoming profoundly more fatigued and depressed. Where just before the course of Interferon I was still running four miles a day, there were days now that I barely wanted to get out of bed.

It was at this point that I finally realized what was going to happen to me—I was going to die. From the first moment of that realization to this very day, it is not the act of passing from life to death that frightens me, but the events up to that point. The body and the physical abilities of which I had been so proud, and for which I had worked so hard, are deteriorating with cancer and weakness.

There is virtually nothing I can do or say that will change this situation much. I have been part of four different protocols, or experimental treatments, and have shown improvement on three of them. However, my progress was not sufficient to warrant continuation of any of them.

The Shanti Project

The Shanti Project in San Francisco delivers the types of services most needed by people with AIDS. It is a nonprofit organization that provides free volunteer assistance and counseling on a long-term basis to patients facing life-threatening illnesses. As of September 1983, the Shanti Project had worked individually with 276 persons with AIDS. The volunteer counselors are a heterogeneous group—many coming from the helping professions and almost all having experienced a personal life-threatening illness or profound loss. They are trained, both academically and experientially, to offer a caring presence to the terminally ill patient. Many of the volunteers have themselves been assisted through the Shanti Project.

In addition to counseling, the Shanti Project supplies community volunteers who give not only support and companionship but also such assistance as transportation, cooking, cleaning, and so forth. By being available to take care of mail, plants, or pets and by visiting or taking favorite food, the volunteers and counselors give a sense of continuity to an unpredictable life, and they extinguish many day-to-day worries with which the person with AIDS may be unable to cope.

Support groups are another important, perhaps vital, resource for people with AIDS offered by the Shanti Project and by similar groups in other cities. Knowing that others face similar problems, fear similar fears, and share similar joys is comforting to each of us—but it is especially necessary for those who are as isolated from society as are many people with AIDS. It is necessary to note, however, that some people with AIDS are unable to face their peers and the reality of their own illness. Watching others whom we learn to care about slowly waste away or suddenly die is extremely traumatic, but the realization for people with AIDS that they are also watching themselves can be too much to handle.

Coordinating Efforts

In San Francisco it is not unusual for people with AIDS to receive services through community health programs or independent providers, as well as assistance from the Shanti Project counselors and community volunteers. However, many volunteer counselors are not trained to handle the complicated problems that arise when suicidal thoughts or severe psychopathology, such as psychotic symptoms, appear. Mental health professionals are needed because they are trained to diagnose and treat the more severe psychological problems that may require medication or hospitalization. Patients need to be referred to community mental health crisis units and to private practice psychiatrists and psychologists. Importantly, these referrals need to be made with care, taking into account the provider's experience with the gay community, understanding of the mental health aspects of AIDS, and receptivity to treating a person with AIDS.

We believe that the needs of people with AIDS cannot be fully met without coordination between community groups and professionals trained in the mental health specialties.

Lovers, Friends, and Family

The mental health aspects of the AIDS crisis affect not only those with AIDS but also the people in their lives. Lovers, friends, and family are all likely to experience significant distress and may need mental health services. Because AIDS is a mysterious and stigmatized illness, the psychological issues raised for significant others may be more complicated than those for other life-threatening illnesses.

We recently spoke with a man whose lover had died of AIDS only 3 weeks before:

The morning of the day that my lover died, I found him looking into a mirror and crying. That was the first time he had realized just how thin he had become. He went through our house to organize it, to set the hangers in the closet "two fingers apart" as he had been taught in military school, to straighten up our bedroom for review. He told me I should take him to the hospital so that I wouldn't have to deal with his body. Once we were there, I went out to call both of our families. He told me: "Don't worry, I'll wait for you." When I came back, I sat by his bed, we held hands, and he died. I guess he decided that it was better that he died rather than suffer through what he knew he would have to face.

Issues of loss and bereavement need to be addressed most carefully for people with AIDS and for their lovers and family. Since most gay men with AIDS are fairly young, their lovers and friends are not as equipped to deal with the issues of death as older people may be. In cities such as New York and San Francisco, where there is a high concentration of AIDS, it is not unusual for someone to have several friends who have been diagnosed. The "unfairness" of dying in an epidemic, and of a disease that has no known cure, is exacerbated by the stigma of being gay, living in atypical relationships, and being avoided by many friends out of fear of contagion. The following paragraphs are one man's reaction after his diagnosis of KS:

All of my mental preparation was insufficient to thwart the tidal wave of emotion that swept over me as I received what, at the time, I regarded as a death sentence. I went home that evening in the company of my lover Michael, feeling the weight of two worlds on my shoulders—mine and his. Wanting to protect him from contracting the disease himself, and from the difficulties that I knew were ahead, I asked him to leave me. He refused.

Michael took the news worse than I, initially. As I look back on those days now, I realize that I didn't have time to think of myself, I was too busy taking care of him. He cried, I guess for about six weeks—to the point that my own emotion had to be contained. Eventually, though, we were able to cry together. It has not been easy allowing myself the relief—the freedom—that such crying brings.

For those of you with friends with AIDS, please remember that this is no time for an "out of sight, out of mind" philosophy. When one of your friends is too ill to participate in your life as they did before, don't just forget them. Remember, this is when they need you the most. If you can, respond to that need.

The lovers of persons with AIDS have special psychological needs. Knowing that one has shared the most intimate contact with another who is dying of a contagious disease can be shattering, and the extent of knowledge about AIDS is such that medical evidence cannot fully dispel these fears. Once more is known about contagion and specific patient characteristics associated with susceptibility, many of these men may feel personally more at ease. Although this group has not been adequately studied, it does not appear that most lovers of people with AIDS have developed the syndrome. Unfortunately, lovers of people with AIDS have more reasons for developing emotional problems than concern over their own health: they are almost certain to face self-righteousness, discrimination, fear, and legal impediments as they help their lover through the last months or years of his life. These are psychological demands that pile atop existing grief and health worries, and they suggest the need for mental health and support services.

When people are diagnosed with AIDS, their friends are faced with a series of distressing issues. Gay friends may be particularly vulnerable because they can readily identify with their friend. Indeed, friends often over-identify and act as if they have just been diagnosed. Other reactions include awkwardness in discussing the illness and problems in working through their fears regarding contagion. Some people want to be supportive, but may not know how to do so. For many, the diagnosis of a friend leads to existential questions and difficult reappraisals of their own lifestyle. For heterosexual friends who may not have known of the person's sexual orientation, the situation may be similarly awkward.

Families of gay men with AIDS have reactions similar to those of close friends. For some, diagnosis brings with it disclosure of a life-threatening illness as well as disclosure of sexual orientation. Families that do not accept the homosexuality of a person going through such a difficult period are likely to experience considerable difficulty. The social stigma of the diagnosis involves a presumption about the person's lifestyle that is a source of stress, and the stigma further complicates the family's bereavement.

The Shanti Project reported that as of mid-September of 1983, 632 lovers, friends, or family members of people with AIDS have been given individual counseling. This total is well over twice as many people served as those with AIDS. Thus, each new case of AIDS diagnosed in the country has a ripple effect, increasing the need for mental health services. To our knowledge, no data have yet been gathered about the impact of AIDS on the demand for mental health services in either the public or private sectors, but it is clear that mental health services that are AIDS-related are needed in cities that have a large number of people with AIDS.

The Gray Zone

If AIDS is caused by an infectious agent, it seems reasonable that the agent would produce a spectrum of illnesses ranging from subclinical to fatal. The current definition of AIDS used by the Centers for Disease Control (CDC) requires the presence of a disease (for example, KS, PCP, or other serious opportunistic infection) at least moderately indicative of defective cell-mediated immunity in a person who has no known cause to account for such a defect. A large group of patients can be identified who manifest less well-defined symptoms of immune deficiency. This condition has been variously referred to as pre-AIDS, prodromal AIDS, or lesser AIDS. One man in this group referred to his experience as "life in the gray zone."

Some people report no symptoms but have laboratory evidence of immune deficiency. Some report nonspecific symptoms of fever, weight loss, and chronic lymphadenopathy. Some have such diseases as oral candidiasis and various forms of herpes. One man who has been at the more severe end of this spectrum for almost 2 years reports the following:

I guess I'm luckier than most of the "victims." I've been sick almost 24 months now, and my wife and good friends are still here. I have new friends. My prognosis looks better. Beta-strep was my last infection, but that was over 3 months ago and I haven't been seriously ill since. They now tell me that I definitely do not have CDC-defined AIDS.

I suppose I should feel relieved, yet because of current research findings, I am treated with even greater precautions than ever before. Regardless of what I do have, I'm still in the NIH AIDS Study Group, examined only in "AIDS Precautions" rooms, and now for the first time in 24 months my blood is drawn by a masked, capped, gloved, and gowned mummy.

It is important to note that I no longer have the same sense of fear—I'm not among the 80 percent of AIDS patients who will die. Yet, the emotional trauma and the social judgments were as real as theirs.

No one should have to experience that journey alone, without help.

There is disagreement on how best to meet the mental health needs of this group. Most professionals believe that supportive psychotherapy—supplying empathy and a nonjudgmental atmosphere in which to discuss any issue—can greatly lower levels of distress. Some researchers and clinicians believe that stress plays an important role in both susceptibility and progression of AIDS, based on findings in psychoimmunology that show a quantifiable relationship between emotional distress and specific immune system functioning.

Those suggesting a relationship between stress and immune functioning would argue for active interventions to reduce stress for people with evidence of immune suppression. Biofeedback, relaxation training, hypnosis, or any other techniques designed to teach coping mechanisms for reducing stress could be used. The argument is that some of these people could show increased resistance to illness as a result of practicing stress reduction techniques. This is clearly an area for future research.

The Worried Well

AIDS anxiety has struck gay men across the country, including many without reason to be particularly fearful. These men interpret every cough as PCP, look for KS lesions on their bodies several times a day, and dread minor infections that they are sure will turn into a life-threatening illness. A physician told us:

> We are seeing a series of people who, even though they had been tested as much as people test for this, insist on being tested again. No one will give them another screening because they have just had one. They are very anxious and agitated and sometimes depressed, having trouble with work, having trouble with roommates and lovers, all because of this concern. They keep saying: "What's my risk? Do I have it or not? I want another test."

Those who fall into this group are often referred to as the "worried well." These medically asymptomatic gay men have developed psychological symptoms that include actual panic attacks, generalized anxiety, hypochondriasis, and somatic preoccupation. Often these episodes involve unfounded beliefs that one is actually dying of AIDS. In other cases, episodes involve obsessional thinking about disease. These AIDS-related anxiety states can be sufficiently severe to impair social and occupational functioning.

The worried well can often be assisted by supplying accurate information about AIDS. However, a proportion of this group will require more specific assessment, diagnosis, and treatment. In other cases, stress reduction techniques have proved to be of assistance in treating anxiety symptoms. Many of these people benefit most from traditional psychotherapy that uses uncovering approaches designed to resolve conflicts that have been brought to the surface by the threat of AIDS.

The Gay Community

Gay males in general are at high risk for mental health problems because of the AIDS epidemic. The frustrations related to being gay in a nonunderstanding society are magnified by a new and pervasive fear of AIDS. Public attacks against people with AIDS as "immoral homosexuals" who have reaped the rewards for their sins do have an effect on people's minds. Gay males are not unaware that 70 to 75 percent of persons with AIDS are gay males, and this fact gives rise to considerable worry.

As the AIDS crisis worsens, gay men are becoming more concerned. A survey of gay men in San Francisco in March 1983 found that approximately 75 percent of the respondents indicated increased anxiety since they had found out about AIDS. Denial of the problems associated with AIDS was low—only 3 percent agreed with the statement that one need not worry because a cure was forthcoming. Only 8 percent of the respondents felt that they had heard too much about AIDS, and only 7 percent indicated that AIDS had not affected them at all.

Gay community organizations in the most heavily affected cities have developed programs to deal with the anxieties that gay men have regarding AIDS. Some of these organizations offer "worried well" support groups, with the goals of information sharing and support for health-conscious behaviors. AIDS awareness workshops and AIDS phone hotlines are also offered for people to discuss their concerns about AIDS and suggest coping strategies. In addition, many gay organizations have developed and distributed AIDS risk-reduction guidelines. We see an absolute need for cooperation among these gay community agencies and city or county health departments, city or county mental health departments, and providers of mental health services who are in private practice.

The fact that gay organizations are becoming increasingly involved with AIDS as a health and mental health issue illustrates a crucial point. There is real, not just imagined, discrimination against gay people in health care settings and from health care professionals—be it active or passive. Gay men with AIDS have been told that their lovers may not see them in intensive care units—when hospital policy prohibits anyone but "family members" from visiting. Hospital procedures do not allow for a same-sex spouse to take responsibility for an incapacitated patient. Health care workers are often shocked to see two men care for each other so deeply, and it takes time and patience on all sides before the realization dawns that these gay men are no different, yet oddly set apart, from the rest of society.

While it is unrealistic to expect every physician to understand, recognize, and be able to treat all known health problems, it is too often the case that gay-related problems are effectively overlooked or clearly misdiagnosed. Mental health professionals do not necessarily have better or sufficient understanding of the particular issues that lesbians and gay males face. As a consequence, gay-oriented health clinics and social service centers have been formed in those few cities that can support such an operation. These centers serve an important function, but they also lessen the demand on traditional health care professionals to expand their understanding of gay issues.

Although public health agencies have not been outspoken on the topic of assuring appropriate health care services for gay men, this is changing as a result of AIDS. The editor of Morbidity and Mortality Weekly Report, published by the Centers for Disease Control, has written: "The classification of certain groups as being more closely associated with the disease (AIDS) has been misconstrued by some to mean these groups are likely to transmit the disease through non-intimate interactions. This view is not justified by available data. Nonetheless, it has been used unfairly as a basis for social and economic discrimination."

There are psychological ramifications to these stigmas. Someone who is seriously ill is virtually unable to cope with overcoming pervasive homophobia in a hospital staff. Depression over being hospitalized can be counted on to worsen when the person is faced with discriminatory treatment as well. Insensitivity by a few staff members can interfere with extremely positive attitudes of all others.

Clearly, there is a proper role for public health agencies in fighting this discrimination. Staff of health departments and mental health centers can add new, important voices to the out-cry. They can sponsor public education programs, work with the gay communities to reduce risk, and intervene with hospitals and professional groups to promote the best possible care for gay men faced with this terrifying epidemic.

Health Professionals

As in any crisis, the AIDS epidemic has brought out many ex-tremely dedicated health care providers. These physicians, nurses, orderlies, psychologists, social workers, and social service workers have spent unprecedented amounts of time helping peo-ple in need. But the new "specialists" in AIDS are at risk for emo-tional distress. Floundering with experimental treatments for an uncertain disease, and losing patient after patient, again and again, is difficult. Being one of the few practitioners in an area who has any understanding of AIDS, and believing that if you do not see this next person perhaps no one else can, leads to personal expectations that are impossible to meet as the AIDS crisis grows. The director of a mental health crisis unit told us:

In the initial phase when I was doing a lot of crisis intervention my-self, I would call back the referring person to lament and bemoan what had happened to a 30-year-old man just diagnosed with AIDS. It's about as touching and full of pathos as any situation that I could think of. And then we're called on to go to the next one, to the next one, to the next one . . .

Beyond issues of overwork and burnout, health care profes-sionals are faced with special problems associated with AIDS. An-ger is a major part in the lives of most people with AIDS that we know, and this anger is often directed at the practitioner who can-not answer questions, who cannot offer hope, but who counsels participation in yet another experimental procedure for a cure. AIDS is also a political issue; practitioners need to be careful of what they say and how they approach their patients. The specter of political repression for homosexual activity and fears that pa-tient confidentiality will be breached lead patients to demand that their diagnosis not be reported to public health agencies, and this demand brings up ethical problems which must be addressed. The glare of publicity for AIDS-related work can be a burden as well, particularly when requests for media interviews begin to interfere with professional and personal time.

The mental health needs of health care professionals working with AIDS should be a cause for increased concern. Traditional ways of dealing with burnout, such as taking vacations, still work, and these responses need to be relearned. Other techniques may need to be encouraged. The directors of many agencies where there is a high level of stress insist on weekly staff meetings where cases are discussed and, more importantly, individual staff members have an opportunity to discuss personal reactions. Health care providers working with AIDS appear to need either formal or informal ways of talking about their experiences in a supportive environment. Unless time is set aside to discuss these issues, symptoms of distress are likely to develop rapidly.

The psychological problems facing gay professionals who are dealing with AIDS are immensely complex. Many will over-identify with people with AIDS and push themselves too hard. Certainly, some who are confronted with AIDS patients tend to resurface their own fears of AIDS and may become part of the "worried well." Others have special fears of contagion. The many gay practitioners who are not self-identified are faced with fears of backlash if it comes out that they are homosexual, and the anxiety over possible loss of job and status, merely on the basis of being identified as gay, can be overwhelming. Those who accept being gay, and who work in an environment that is accepting, can build a special network of friends and colleagues who will be supportive. Those who must avoid such public knowledge, for personal or professional reasons, are at high risk for emotional distress unless they have a way to vent and work through their frustrations.

Conclusion

Individuals are reacting to the threat of an unknown but deadly epidemic with fear when strength is needed, with denial when awareness is needed, with guilt when understanding is needed, and with withdrawal when caring is needed. We believe that it is the responsibility of the health and mental health community, as broadly defined, to respond to the psychological needs of persons with AIDS and to the needs of their lovers and families.

Over time, more progress will be made in understanding, treating, and preventing AIDS. If, as it appears, AIDS strikes with varying degrees of severity, many people will undergo the physical and emotional turmoil and live to tell about it. Still others will die, deeply bitter at knowing that the cure will come too late. Many more will be affected by the fear of the disease, and by the suffering of friends, family, or lovers with AIDS. The psychological impact of AIDS is likely to remain for a long, long time.

THE PURSUIT OF A CURE[4]

AIDS invariably kills. Each year the number of victims suffering from acquired immune deficiency syndrome doubles, and the plague has spread far beyond the homosexual community where doctors diagnosed the first cases in 1981. Scientists are searching for ways to combat AIDS but the prognosis for patients is no better than it was four years ago: most will die within three years of contracting the condition. There is still no effective vaccine—or even effective treatment—against the AIDS virus. And the most recent discoveries, while producing important new insights, are chilling. Last March scientists at the National Institutes of Health (NIH) in Bethesda, Md., discovered that AIDS, which depresses the body's immune system weakening its ability to resist infection, also attacks and kills brain cells. And last month U.S. researchers learned that AIDS viral cells reproduce faster than any other known virus. Concluded William Haseltine, a molecular biologist at Harvard University: "At this point, in the battle between man and microbe we are definitely losing."

Researchers and clinicians now have only two ways of attacking AIDS: by attempting to kill the virus—or at least stopping it from reproducing, and by strengthening the patient's ravaged immune system. HPA-23, a substance developed at the Pasteur Institute in Paris, has received widespread attention since actor Rock Hudson flew there in the hope that the antiviral drug would

[4]Reprint of an article by Pat Ohlendorf, *Maclean's*. Reprinted by permission from *Maclean's*, 98:36–7. Ag. 12, '85. Copyright © 1985 by *Maclean's*.

help his condition. But it is only one of several similar compounds, including Suramin, which was used as long ago as 1920 to arrest African sleeping sickness. Those drugs have shown some promise in animal research but so far the results obtained after tests on humans have been inconclusive. NIH scientist Robert Gallo, co-discoverer of the AIDS virus, declared that faith in HPA-23 might prove to be unfounded: "I am a little put off by the publicity centred on one compound which I would not call very outstanding."

In fact, the aim of many clinical researchers is to determine how well current antiviral drugs—none of which is commercially available—react on different patients. Gallo's group is investigating Suramin, and a group of Montreal physicians also wants to begin testing that compound, as well as Foscarnet. Almost everyone involved with those drugs—researchers, doctors or even representatives of the pharmaceutical firms producing the substances—say that it is far too early to gauge their effectiveness. Said Dr. Roger Fontaine, medical director of the French firm that produces HPA-23: "We think it may have some influence on the virus that causes AIDS but we are far from sure that we have a drug to cure it." Added Dr. Norbert Gilmore, a Montreal immunologist and chairman of the National Advisory Committee on AIDS: "Some of these substances clearly stop the virus from replicating, at least while the drug is administered. But that may not mean a cure." Once patients stop taking drugs the virus renews its rapid proliferation. As well, antiviral treatments often produce such serious side effects as liver damage and loss of blood-clotting ability.

Unabated: Most scientists trying to defeat AIDS by building up the body's immune system with such drugs as interferon and interleukin have failed. The virus continues replicating unabated despite the treatments. Even radical attempts to replace, or at least build up, the body's failed immune system through bone marrow and thymus gland transplants have been unsuccessful because the virus simply kills the new T-helper cells—white blood cells that direct the body's resistance to infection. Declared Donald Abrams, assistant director of the San Francisco General Hospital's AIDS clinic: "Ultimately, we will probably need a combination of both therapies." And physicians still do not know which combination of antiviral and immune system builders would best help AIDS victims. Indeed, Gilmore's description of

AIDS treatment at Montreal's Royal Victoria Hospital could be applied to any AIDS clinic in the world. Said Gilmore: "Most of the work we do is counselling."

At the same time, there does not appear to be any imminent breakthrough in finding an effective vaccine to prevent AIDS. In fact, researchers do not know whether it will ever be possible to create a vaccine, because the virus—called HTLV-III in North America and LAV in France—might be mutating, or changing its characteristics, so rapidly that it could prove to be an elusive target. And if it is possible, a workable vaccine would first have to be tested thoroughly. As a result, cautioned molecular biologist Flossie Wong-Staal, a member of Dr. Gallo's team, such a vaccine might not be ready for the public for "a couple of years." But by that time nearly 50,000 more Americans and 1,200 more Canadians will have AIDS, and 25,000 North Americans will have died from the disease.

Register: AIDS is such a new phenomenon that even present methods of diagnosis are sometimes inadequate. A small and still-unknown percentage of people infected by AIDS show negative results when their blood is tested for the condition. The reason: the current tests used to detect the disease measure antibodies that the body manufactures to fight the virus; those victims may have so many more AIDS virus cells than antibodies that the antibodies simply do not register on the test. As well, a test that could detect the virus rather than the body's reaction to the virus has still not been developed. Said Wong-Staal: "It is like looking for a needle in a haystack. If you take tissue from any given person, only one in 1,000—or even one in 10,000—cells will be infected by the virus."

Still, scientific work is continuing at a feverish pace in North American and European laboratories to understand the AIDS virus thoroughly. Without that knowledge, searches for a vaccine and for effective treatments cannot succeed. So far, researchers have determined that the virus is made up of six genes, and they have learned the functions of only four of them. One of them is highly unusual. The tiny gene triggers the virus to reproduce at an incredible speed. Said Haseltine: "We can now explain why the AIDS virus holds the world's record. It replicates 10 to 100 times faster than any other we know about—it's really a heavyweight." That not only demonstrates how rapidly the virus may be mutating—because, said Haseltine, "rapid replication means more mistakes in copying genetic instructions"—but it also suggested that only a tiny amount of the virus may be needed to infect a new victim.

But Wong-Staal, for one, still says that finding an effective vaccine may be possible. Added the researcher: "We should not play up the negative implications of this until we have actually tried the vaccine experiments." Haseltine even holds out the prospect of "using the nastiness of the virus against itself"—using the newly discovered gene to trigger rapid manufacture of substances to treat or prevent AIDS.

AIDS also has a powerful ability to kill brain cells. Doctors initially noticed that some victims were depressed, had trouble grasping new concepts or were behaving strangely. Some physicians attributed those symptoms to the shock of adjusting to the death sentence that AIDS imposes and others said that the changes were caused by brain tumors. But Gallo's researchers made a further discovery when they dissected brain tissue taken from 15 patients who had died. In one-third of the cases they found that the virus had directly attacked the brain cells. In fact, the brains of young children who die of AIDS are sometimes one-third smaller than brains of healthy children at the same age, indicating that the AIDS virus either arrests brain development or destroys cerebral tissue. But for most adult AIDS victims, brain disease is not a major concern. They are aware that they are much more likely to succumb to secondary infections of an especially virulent pneumonia, Kaposi's sarcoma or cancer tumors long before the virus causes fatal brain disease.

Concern: Some doctors—increasingly discouraged as they helplessly watch patients die—say that more research is needed on the secondary infections that actually cause death. The concern expressed by Constance Wofsy, specialist in infectious diseases and a co-director of the San Francisco General Hospital's AIDS clinic, underlines the hopelessness many clinicians feel in the face of the mounting AIDS epidemic: "We just don't have enough drugs to treat conditions like the pneumonia, Kaposi's or the cytomegalovirus that leads to blindness. Of course the patients will die anyway, but we should try harder to increase the amount of time they have left, even if it is only a few months. We should be concentrating on improving the quality of the little life remaining to those patients, to see that they are reasonably comfortable, and that they are able to die with dignity."

AIDS PROGRESS REPORT[5]

Without question, AIDS was the major medical news story of 1985. Unfortunately, media reports of patients traveling to Europe to seek treatment or of victims' friends smuggling drugs into the United States from Mexico have left the impression that efforts to combat this devastating disease are lagging in this country.

The truth is that tremendous progress has been made in AIDS research in a very short time. In fact, research on AIDS has moved further, and sooner, than has been the case with virtually any other fatal or sexually transmitted disease.

The U.S. Public Health Service has marshaled its resources to bring a coordinated attack on the dreaded disease, tracking its course, identifying its cause, seeking a cure, and preventing its spread through the nation's blood supply.

The world became aware of the existence of acquired immunodeficiency syndrome, or AIDS, in July 1981, when the U.S. Centers for Disease Control first described the syndrome in its *Morbidity and Mortality Weekly Report.* In the more than four years that have followed that event, much has been learned about AIDS. The basic facts are these:

AIDS is a complex disease caused by a virus known as HTLV-III. The initials stand for "human T-cell lymphotrophic virus type III." Identified by scientists at the National Institutes of Health and in France (where it is called lymphadenopathy associated virus, or LAV), HTLV-III is one of a family of retroviruses associated with human diseases.

HTLV-III attacks certain cells that play a key role in the human immune system, leaving patients vulnerable to a variety of "opportunistic" infections, such as pneumonia caused by the organism *Pneumocystis carinii* and a rare form of cancer called Kaposi's sarcoma.

By the end of 1985, more than 14,500 cases of AIDS had been reported nationwide; about half of these patients have died. AIDS has been reported from all 50 states as well as other countries.

[5]Reprint of an article by Annabel Hecht, member of FDA's public affairs staff. Reprinted by permission from *FDA Consumer*, 20:32-5. F. '86.

AIDS is usually spread by sexual contact. About 70 percent of AIDS victims have been sexually active homosexual or bisexual men. Heterosexual contacts of AIDS patients or of persons at high risk for AIDS can also develop the disease.

The virus can also be transmitted by blood from infected persons. Intravenous drug users are at high risk when they share needles. A small percentage of AIDS cases have resulted from transfusions of blood or of certain blood products such as those needed by hemophiliacs.

A laboratory test has been developed that can detect the presence of antibodies to the HTLV-III virus in blood and plasma. Approved by FDA early in 1985, the test is being used by the nation's blood banks to screen out any blood and plasma that may be a source of AIDS. (See "Screening Blood Donations for AIDS" in the May 1985 *FDA Consumer.*)

The new test, plus new methods to render harmless any viruses that may be present in blood products used by hemophiliacs, should prevent transmission of AIDS by this route.

AIDS also has been reported in infants whose mothers had the disease or were associated with AIDS patients. Usually, it is not known whether the virus was transmitted from mother to child before, during or shortly after birth.

Present evidence indicates that the average person who is not in a high-risk group and has no intimate contact with high-risk individuals has no reason to worry about getting AIDS. All available data suggest that the disease is not spread by casual, everyday contact with infected persons. Donating blood in no way exposes the donor to AIDS since disposable equipment is used.

The incubation period for AIDS—from the time the virus enters the body to the onset of the disease—is not absolutely known, although studies have shown it is usually several months to two and a half years but can be longer than five years. A person exposed to the virus may never develop AIDS but may be a carrier. About 20 percent of exposed individuals develop less severe symptoms of AIDS, a condition called AIDS-related complex.

Once a person has developed AIDS, the prospect of recovery is dim; no victim has been known to survive. There is no known cure or treatment for AIDS. No scientist anywhere in the world has ever claimed to have discovered a cure.

Because of the complexity of the disease, the search for an effective AIDS treatment has had to move in three directions at once: (1) finding and testing drugs that will stop the growth of HTLV-III; (2) developing a means of rebuilding the victim's immune system; and (3) improving the treatment of the rare cancers and opportunistic infections that follow the breakdown of the immune system.

Further compounding the difficulty in finding a cure for AIDS is the fact that anti-viral research is a relatively new field of science. Few drugs are available to combat *any* viruses. Isolating and measuring viruses in body fluids is extremely difficult, time-consuming and expensive.

The problem lies in the nature of viruses. Unlike free-living bacteria, which have the capability to multiply on their own, viruses can only reproduce inside living cells. Viruses carry their own genetic code but need biochemical functions provided by the "host" cell to produce new viruses. HTLV-III has a particular liking for a subclass of lymphocytes called T-4 cells, blood cells that are responsible for initiating and regulating immune functions in the human body. (See "How the Body Fights for Its Health" in the April 1983 *FDA Consumer.*)

One approach to AIDS treatment is to disrupt the life cycle of the virus; a major hurdle is finding a compound that will kill the virus or infected host cells without destroying uninfected host cells.

A number of compounds with the potential for interfering with viral replication are under clinical investigation, including suramin, ribavirin, azidothymidine, HPA-23 and phosphonoformate.

Suramin, an anti-parasite drug made by Bayer AG (a West German firm), has been used to treat African sleeping sickness and river blindness. Soon after the discovery of the AIDS virus, laboratory tests showed that the drug could block growth of the virus and inhibit its ability to kill T-4 cells. Suramin was found to suppress the virus's growth temporarily in a small number of patients in a National Institutes of Health study, but it had significant side effects, including kidney failure and liver damage. So far, it has produced little or no clinical benefit, but studies are continuing to determine if more extended treatment may be of value.

Ribavirin has also shown an ability to inhibit the growth of HTLV-III in the laboratory. The drug has been used experimentally in infants in aerosol form for infections caused by respirato-

ry syncytial virus. Side effects seen from the dosage given in
aerosol form appear thus far to be minimal. But side effects in
AIDS patients in a few studies conducted at university hospitals
in the United States, in which the drug is given in higher doses
and in oral or intravenous form, have included severe anemia. Vi-
ratek, Inc., a subsidiary of ICN Pharmaceuticals of California, is
planning clinical trials of an oral dosage form.

Another antiviral approved for experimental testing in this
country is azidothymidine, made by the Burroughs Wellcome Co.
of North Carolina. Laboratory studies conducted at FDA and at
the National Cancer Institute show that the drug can inhibit the
ability of HTLV-III to infect immune cells and to reproduce. Initial safety studies, under way at the National Institutes of Health
and Duke University, appear to confirm some of the laboratory
findings, although additional studies are needed to determine if
there are clinical benefits. Side effects are minimal or absent at
doses currently being tested.

Of the drugs being studied to combat AIDS, the one which
is probably most well known to the public is HPA-23, the French
drug reportedly used by Rock Hudson and sought by many other
AIDS victims. HPA-23 had been reported to inhibit growth of
HTLV-III in the laboratory; however, when it was used on 47 patients at the Pasteur Institute in France, no clinical improvement
was shown. Adverse reactions included a decrease in the platelet
count, bleeding, liver damage and abdominal pain. In the United
States, studies have begun at five medical centers to evaluate the
toxicity and to determine the effects of the drug on the virus in
patients. Also, treatment of a small number of Americans who received the drug on a chronic basis in France have begun at two
other medical centers. HPA-23 is produced by the drug firm
Rhône-Poulenc.

Phosphonoformate, also called PFA or Foscarnet, is another
anti-viral drug that has been shown to inhibit replication of the
AIDS virus in laboratory studies. PFA is also known to have activity against several herpes viruses that cause some of the severe opportunistic infections that strike AIDS patients. Clinical trials of
PFA are under way in Denmark and Sweden. The major known
side effect is kidney damage.

Another approach to AIDS treatment is to try to rebuild the
patient's damaged immune system. As AIDS progresses, the
virus spreads from one cell to another in a process of "internal
contagion."

It is believed that the immune system may regenerate either spontaneously or with therapeutic help if action is taken before too many T-4 cells are destroyed. (Unfortunately, one characteristic of retroviruses is that they can become incorporated into the genetic material of the host cell, lie dormant, and be reactivated at a later time.)

Among the immune system "enhancers" under study is interleukin-2, a protein produced by normal lymphocytes in response to viral infections. Early laboratory studies by FDA scientists indicated that interleukin-2 increased the activity of lymphocytes from AIDS patients. A few patients among 35 treated with interleukin-2 during a two-year study experienced improvement in their immune systems. No clinical improvement was seen in their overall condition, however. The drug has been produced by various manufacturers, such as Hoffmann-La Roche, Cetus Corp., and Collaborative Research Inc.

Isoprinosine has been reported to enhance some aspects of the immune response in patients with AIDS-related complex (ARC). Made by Newport Pharmaceuticals of Newport, Calif., isoprinosine was studied at St. Luke's Roosevelt Hospital in New York City in a small group of patients with AIDS and ARC. However, the studies failed to show effectiveness in the treatment of AIDS and only minimal effects in some laboratory tests of immune function in a few patients with ARC. A New Drug Application for isoprinosine is under review at FDA for treatment of ARC and persistent generalized lymphadenopathy, another milder form of HTLV-III infection.

Another drug reported to stimulate the immune system is IMREG-1, made by IMREG Inc. of New Orleans. IMREG-1 will be used at the M.D. Anderson Hospital in Dallas and a number of other locations to study its effect in patients with ARC. Thus far, there is no indication of any clinical effects.

Scientists at the National Institute of Allergy and Infectious Diseases are investigating the effects of bone marrow transplantation in three AIDS patients. The patients have received transplants from their healthy identical twins. This treatment is being combined with transfusion of lymphocytes from the healthy twin and administration of the anti-viral drug suramin.

French investigators recently claimed dramatic improvements in some functions of the immune systems in patients given cyclosporine, a drug approved by FDA in 1983 to prevent rejection of organ transplants. However, these findings were very preliminary and some of the patients under treatment have died. Following the initial announcement, Sandoz Pharmaceuticals, manufacturer of cyclosporine under the brand name Sandimmune, announced plans to sponsor clinical trials to determine whether the drug may play a role in the treatment of AIDS.

Treatments are also being sought for the "opportunistic" infections that are so often devastating for AIDS victims. While a healthy person would be able to fight these infections, the weakened immune system of AIDS patients allows the infections to run rampant with sometimes lethal force. Treating these complications does not change the course of AIDS but may improve the quality of the patient's life.

One of the most prevalent of these infections is *Pneumocystis carinii* pneumonia, which develops in about 60 percent of AIDS patients. Trimethoprim/sulfamethoxazole, a prescription combination drug also used to treat urinary tract infections and ear infections in children, and pentamidine isethionate are generally effective, although they cause severe reactions in about half the patients.

Many AIDS patients have progressive cytomegalovirus (CMV) infections that can lead to inflammation of the retina, blindness, colitis, pneumonia and death. A number of investigators at NIH and FDA are collaborating on a study to test 9-(1,3, dehydroxy-2-propoxymethyl) guanine (DHPG) in the treatment of severe CMV infections. DHPG has shown temporary activity against CMV in a small number of patients.

At Cornell University Medical College in New York City, researchers are studying the effectiveness of gamma interferon in treating patients with *Mycobacterium avium intracellulare* infections that affect the respiratory tract.

Experimental treatments for Kaposi's sarcoma include agents such as alpha-interferon, chemotherapy and radiation therapy.

At the Medical College of Virginia, researchers are comparing the effectiveness of two marketed anti-fungal drugs, 5-fluorocytosine and amphotericin B, as treatments for AIDS patients with opportunistic fungal infections.

At St. Vincent's Hospital and Medical Center in New York, researchers are studying the efficacy of a range of antibiotics in treating patients with cryptosporidiosis, an infection that causes severe, protracted diarrhea and weight loss. The antiparasitic drug alpha-difluoro-methyl-ornithine (DFMO) is being tested against this illness at the General Clinical Research Center at Cornell University Medical College.

FDA has expedited all requests for the study of experimental agents for AIDS and has met with all manufacturers, including those in Europe, who have expressed an interest in submitting an application to test a new drug. In several instances, potentially useful compounds have gained "orphan drug" status, which provides financial incentives, including tax benefits, to sponsors for drugs that may not result in much financial return. Among the AIDS drugs with orphan status are pentamidine, HPA-23, azidothymidine and DHPG.

At times there has been criticism that FDA's regulations hold up availability of vital treatment for AIDS patients. However, the importance of controlled clinical trials cannot be overemphasized, particularly in the case of a poorly understood disease, such as AIDS. Only a few of the compounds being tested appear to be potentially useful in treating AIDS or its complications and, at this point, no one knows whether some of these compounds might also have a potential for harm, possibly speeding the growth of the virus and shortening the patient's life.

Medical history has shown that the best way to prevent the spread of infectious diseases is through vaccination. Research on a vaccine against AIDS is under way at NIH, where a number of novel approaches are being explored, including several that involve recombinant DNA technology. FDA virologists are working with NIH scientists in the search for an AIDS vaccine.

AIDS patients who wish to participate in clinical trials of experimental AIDS therapies should contact their physicians. Patients should keep in mind that these experimental treatments have not been proven safe and effective but *may* be found worthwhile as a result of such studies.

'FAST-BUCK' ARTISTS ARE MAKING A KILLING ON AIDS[6]

They travel to Tijuana by car, bus, and chartered airplane from as far away as New York City. Thousands of victims of AIDS—and many more who fear that they have contracted the deadly disease—are flocking to the Mexican border town, where they can legally purchase drugs that are experimental in the U.S. On a recent weekend a single planeload of victims from San Francisco spent more than $40,000.

Until some still unforeseen breakthrough is made, hope—and rapidly thinning wallets—is all most victims of acquired immune deficiency syndrome have. So those who have contracted the disease are eager purchasers of unproven drugs and easy prey for quacks, peddlers of questionable treatments—even psychic healers. "Just about anybody who wants to make a fast buck is becoming connected with AIDS," says Morris Kight, a gay-rights activist and member of the County of Los Angeles Human Relations Commission. "It's America's newest fast-growth industry."

Indeed, AIDS may already have created a multibillion-dollar market. Sales of diagnostic tests to screen the blood supply for the AIDS virus will top $150 million worldwide in 1986. And nursing care for AIDS patients sells at premium prices. One clinic in Mexico offers "state of the art" treatment for $20,000 a month. Another in a French chateau will accept a limited number of patients for "lifetime treatment" at $100,000. Medical expenses for AIDS patients are estimated to average $125,000.

Dim Prospects. And the number of cases is still growing. By Nov. 1 the Centers for Disease Control in Atlanta had counted 14,313 cases in the U.S. In addition, it estimates that 500,000 to 1.5 million Americans have been exposed to the virus. As many as 10% of those are developing a mild form of the disease; eventually, many of them may get full-blown AIDS. "There's a lot of business out there," Dr. Timothy J. Dondereo Jr., a CDC epidemiologist, observes wryly.

[6]Reprint of an article by Scott Ticer, *Business Week* staffwriter. Reprinted from December 2, 1985 issue of *Business Week* by special permission, © 1985 by McGraw-Hill, Inc.

Phillip E. Chisum, a 34-year-old Los Angeles computer programmer, is typical of many AIDS patients. Since August, when his doctors told him that he had an early form of the disease, he has paid more than $10,000 for medical care. But he has also taken a drug purchased in Tijuana by a friend and, like many of his friends with AIDS, has considered acupuncture, exercise therapy, or taking huge amounts of vitamins, herbs, and food supplements. What helps the most, he says, is the "metaphysical healer" to whom he's paying $1,140 to focus Chisum's attention on being well. Nonetheless, says Chisum: "The business of AIDS infuriates me. People are making megabucks from a disease."

The search for drugs to stem the inevitably fatal disease is escalating. Drug companies are spending millions, and Congress nearly doubled spending for AIDS research—to $200 million—in the 1986 fiscal year. A dozen drugs are in clinical testing. But people with AIDS aren't willing to wait and see if those drugs will be approved by the Food & Drug Administration.

With dim prospects of being selected for controlled tests, desperate victims are streaming across the Mexican border to buy two experimental drugs: isoprinosine, produced by Newport Pharmaceuticals International Inc., and ICN Pharmaceuticals Inc.'s ribavirin. Both are sold legally there without a prescription.

Behind the rush are abundant—but largely undocumented—testimonials from AIDS victims who say they have benefited from the drugs. Confronted with accusations from homosexual groups that the government is moving too slowly in making the drugs available, the FDA has not opposed the traffic from Mexico, and border agents generally look the other way. A $2 pamphlet distributed by some AIDS organizations details how to acquire, use, and even smuggle the medications.

Luxury Care. Many doctors debunk the effectiveness of the two drugs against AIDS, however. "We have no idea what any of these are going to do against AIDS," worries Dr. Richard C. Straube, an assistant professor at the University of California San Diego Medical Center. Even so, doctors treating AIDS cases on the West Coast estimate that 25% to 30% of the patients they see have tried one or both. ICN says that sales of ribavirin in Mexico have soared 70% this year.

Like the late Rock Hudson, well-heeled victims have additional options. As many as 100 Americans are now being treated in France, where they can more easily obtain experimental drugs.

One new U.S. company is hoping to tap the demand for overseas care. Total Health Enhancement Revitalization Resorts Inc. in Los Angeles claims it has raised $5 million to turn a French chateau into a luxurious AIDS treatment center that will provide— for $100,000—the best medical care available to 20 AIDS patients. "Medical care for the superwealthy is a market that hasn't been touched," explains Genevieve Clavreul, the company's president.

There are also plenty of treatments closer to home. And the proliferation of unverified cures and treatments is starting to attract the attention of law enforcement officials. Last year postal inspectors were granted a temporary restraining order against a Redondo Beach (Calif.) company that was using the mails to pitch a $1,900 "pre-AIDS treatment" in Mexican and West German clinics. In late October the California Dept. of Justice launched its own probe into AIDS frauds. "It's particularly outrageous that these people are becoming victims of medical quackery and health fraud," says Christopher M. Ames, a deputy attorney general who heads the California investigations.

Grim Certainty. "You can get ripped off so easily when you're sick," concedes one AIDS patient. Even so, he paid $250 to a nutritionist and $120 for a telephone consultation with a doctor who recommended massive doses of vitamins. Then an herbalist charged him $50 for a consultation and $100 for herbs. Now he is spending more than $200 a month on vitamins and food supplements.

But until a cure for AIDS is discovered, patients will undoubtedly be easy marks. About the only thing they know for sure is that contracting AIDS means almost certain death—and even that is costing more than usual. Forest Lawn Mortuaries in Los Angeles charges an extra $300 to deal with victims of contagious diseases. "Dying," one AIDS patient points out, "is a business, too."

'LOOK, DOCTOR, I'M DYING. GIVE ME THE DRUG.'[7]

A man finds out that he has a fatal disease. He has about two years left, maybe less. His doctor asks him if he wants to try a new, experimental drug that seems to have helped the first few patients who took it. Sure, the man says. What have I got to lose? Well, the doctor says, we're not sure it works. It may have side effects. It may even make the disease worse. Look, the man says, I know what will happen if you *don't* do anything. Give me the drug.

If you qualify for the clinical trial, the doctor says, you'll have to come to the hospital for a lot of blood tests and different kinds of examinations, and you'll also have to take pills every four hours around the clock, even during the night. And you can't take any other medications unless we say so. Fine, says the man. Give me the drug.

Wait, says the doctor. This is a clinical trial. A double-blind, placebo-controlled, randomized clinical trial. So? says the man. The only way we can find out if the drug really works, says the doctor, is to compare it with no treatment at all: a placebo, a sugar pill. You have a fifty-fifty chance of being assigned at random to the control group, the patients who get the placebo. Neither you nor I will know which you're getting. I don't want a placebo, says the man. Look, doctor, I'm dying. Give me the drug. Leave me out of the clinical trial and just write me a prescription. I'm sorry, says the doctor. The only way to get the drug is to enter the trial.

Variations on this scene have been played out 260 times during the past few months, at a dozen medical centers in eight American cities. The 260 patients have AIDS, and the drug they're testing is AZT, or azidothymidine.* For months, AIDS victims and their families have been calling its manufacturer, the Burroughs Wellcome Co., in Research Triangle Park, N.C., to plead for AZT; some have tried to buy their way into the trial or to bribe employees to get the drug, which Wellcome keeps under lock and key, like a narcotic. One man in the trial says that acquaintances who also have AIDS have told him to hide his bottle

---

[7]Reprint of an article by *Discover* staffwriter Denise Grady. Reprinted by permission from *Discover*, pp. 78–86, Ag. '86. © *Discover* magazine, August '86.
*Its chemical name is 3'-azido-3-deoxythymidine; it's also known as Compound S, and BW A509U.

of capsules when they visit, because they might not be able to resist stealing it. Wellcome declines even to reveal all the entry requirements for the trial, for fear patients will falsify their medical
records to get in. The potential market for AZT, or for any drug
that fights AIDS, is large: 10,000 Americans have the disease,
100,000 have related illnesses caused by the AIDS virus, and a
million and a half more are thought to be carriers. The World
Health Organization estimates there are 50,000 cases of AIDS in
Africa alone, and that 10 million people around the world are infected with the virus.

AZT testing has moved remarkably fast: spokesmen for Wellcome say that in 18 months the drug has arrived at a stage of development that most drugs take four years to reach. The
company, now involved in secret patent negotiations, is investing
$20,000 a patient, for a total of some $5 million, in the trial,
which is scheduled to end in December.

The AZT trial has raised scientific and ethical questions
about medical research on human beings, particularly those who
are dying. It can be difficult to design experiments that treat
these people fairly and at the same time yield the needed information. The ideal experiment would benefit the participants as well
as future patients, but this doesn't always happen, and so one
must ask how much hardship, mental and physical, it's fair to im-
pose on human subjects in the name of research. The current trial, widely regarded as the fastest and most efficient way to test the
drug, is also considered a model for future experiments. But
some scientists have suggested that, without jeopardizing the science, AZT and other drugs meant to fight AIDS could be
dispensed in a more humane way. And they've taken their complaints to Congress. The issue took on added importance on June
30th, when the federal government announced a $100 million
program to test new AIDS drugs, including AZT, at 14 research
centers. The new trials, to include a thousand patients in the first
six months, will also be limited to small groups of patients who
meet specific requirements, and some of them will be given placebos, too.

AZT, an altered form of one of the chemical building blocks
of DNA, was synthesized in 1964 by Jerome Horwitz, a chemist
at the Michigan Cancer Foundation, who thought it might be useful in treating tumors. It wasn't, but when scientists found, late
in 1984, that AIDS was caused by a retrovirus and therefore de-

pended on an unusual enzyme known as reverse transcriptase to reproduce itself, they realized that certain features of the AZT molecule might block that enzyme. Burroughs Wellcome, which is equipped to make the drug but not to work with the AIDS virus, asked Samuel Broder and his colleagues at the National Cancer Institute (NCI) to investigate. Using cultures of AIDS-infected human cells, they showed by February 1985 that AZT didn't kill the virus but did stop it from multiplying. In July they began testing AZT in patients.

In the March 15 issue of the British medical journal *Lancet*, Broder and 17 other scientists cautiously reported that AZT might have made a bit of headway against AIDS. They had given it for six weeks to eleven patients with AIDS and eight with AIDS-related complex, or ARC (which means they were infected with the AIDS virus but had illnesses that didn't fit the official definition of AIDS).

The results, Broder says, were unlike any he had ever encountered. Fifteen patients showed improvements in lab tests that measured the working of their immune systems, two had chronic fungus infections clear up without any other treatment, and six stopped running fevers or having night sweats. In several of the patients who took the highest doses of the drug, cell cultures no longer yielded any traces of the AIDS virus. And although AIDS victims generally waste away, most in the study gained weight: an average of five pounds apiece. Side effects—headaches and lowering of the blood-cell counts, both red and white—weren't severe enough to halt the treatment, except in one case, in which they might have been caused by another drug the patient was taking. AZT crossed the blood-brain barrier, an essential property, because the virus so often attacks the central nervous system. By July 1986, between seven and twelve months after they started taking AZT, 16 of the original 19 patients were still alive. Even though a few had become so anemic that they needed transfusions, most were continuing to use the drug.

As promising as the results were, the scientists considered them good enough only to justify further testing. The first study hadn't even been designed to test AZT's effectiveness but to determine whether it could be tolerated and at what doses. Some of the changes in immune function were small; because AIDS often runs an up-and-down course, and because so few patients were studied for such a short time, it wasn't clear whether the changes were spontaneous or due to the drug. They could also have resulted from the placebo effect, any improvement that occurs simply because a person thinks he ought to feel better because he's being treated; besides, raised spirits may increase the appetite, and eating better may in turn enhance the immune response. Finally, just participating in a study can benefit patients, because they tend to get more medical attention than usual. But even if the gains associated with AZT were real, this first study was too short to predict whether they would last. The virus might somehow develop resistance to the drug. More side effects might emerge with long-term use, or the existing ones might worsen. The researchers insist they don't even know what to make of the fact that so many of the original patients are still alive, because the disease is too unpredictable to assign life expectancies to individuals.

The trial now in progress was designed—mostly by Wellcome, with some help from participating doctors and the Food and Drug Administration (FDA)—to resolve those uncertainties. To qualify, the patients had to have either full-blown AIDS, defined for the purposes of the study as one bout of *Pneumocystis carinii* pneumonia during the previous three months, or ARC. Their results on certain lab tests also had to fall within specific ranges. The idea was to choose subsets of patients so similar to one another that any differences emerging between those treated and the controls could safely be attributed to the drug rather than to differences in the progress of the disease.

After six months the 260 patients are to stop taking their capsules for a month and undergo tests. Wellcome is tabulating the findings, which the twelve treatment centers are submitting continually during the trial. If it's determined that AZT works and is safe, says Dannie King, a microbiologist and Wellcome's AZT project director, "all the patients who participated in the trial will get the drug if they want it." They're protected by several safeguards, he says. First, the original plan may be altered: if there's any indication that a patient would be harmed by withdrawal, the drug won't be taken away, not even for a month. In addition, an independent review board will look at the data every two months during the study, and if one group is faring much better than the other—either because the drug is working wonders or because it's poisoning the subjects—the trial will be halted and all patients will either be offered the drug or taken off it. The first examination of the data will take place in August. "But I can tell you," says King, "it's going to have to be one extraordinary effect to stop that trial."

Wellcome would consider the drug effective, says King, if a statistically significant number of patients improved in the same ways that the original test group did, and if those results were supported by additional gains in overall health and in tests of the immune and nervous systems.

Why, when so many Americans are suffering from AIDS, is this experiment set up to allow only 130 to try such a promising drug? Virtually every researcher interviewed by *Discover*, as well as a spokesman for the FDA, said the drug was in such short supply that there wasn't enough to treat very many more patients. Some blamed a worldwide herring shortage, because herring sperm is one source of the thymidine needed to make AZT.

Pleading scarcity would be an easy out, ethically: you can't deprive people of what you haven't got. This argument can justify the use of placebos, too: it's not that the drug is being withheld deliberately from the controls but that there's not enough for them anyway, and so they're just being studied as a basis for comparison. This is what happened during the field trials of polio vaccine in the summer of 1954, says Robert Levine, a professor of medicine at Yale who also teaches medical ethics and has written a book about clinical trials. Almost 500,000 children received vaccine that summer, while more than a million acted as controls because not enough vaccine could be made for them.

But scarcity, though a problem in the past, is now a false issue, says King. Wellcome is using synthetic thymidine instead of extracting it from herring sperm, and the company could make enough AZT to treat 5,000 people by the end of 1986. But it won't. The number of Americans taking AZT will increase during the next few months, but only to about 1,500, and they will have to enroll in studies at specially designated research centers. Outside these studies, no one can get AZT. It isn't available for "compassionate use," a discretionary category set up by the FDA to allow doctors to prescribe experimental drugs, which must usually be supplied free by the manufacturers, for seriously ill patients. "It's not our charge to manufacture tons of material at great expense, and jeopardize our other clinical programs, just to make sure everybody who wants it can have it," King insists.

The drug is "very, very expensive to make," he says. "I have to provide a stimulus to do this." By which he means solid evidence that the drug works.

The real limiting factor in AZT trials, King says, is ethical. Because the drug may yet prove harmful, the number of patients must be kept small—no larger than needed to provide enough data to stand up to statistical analysis—to minimize the risks. If the company made a single exception for compassionate use, "we couldn't say no to anyone." In that case an unproved drug— possibly worthless or even dangerous—would come into wide-spread use. That, says King, would be unconscionable.

It would also make it virtually impossible to do a placebo-controlled trial: Who would consent to an experiment that offered only a fifty-fifty chance of getting the drug, when requesting it through a doctor would guarantee treatment?

The history of medicine is filled with cautionary tales about unnecessary or harmful treatments that eluded testing, gained acceptance, and hung on for years: radiation therapy for tonsillitis, a brain operation to prevent strokes, a drug for herpes encephalitis that made patients worse, and diethylstilbestrol (DES), an ineffective drug that has caused cancer in the daughters of many women who took it in hopes of preventing miscarriages. Yet if a procedure has become standard practice, and doctors believe in it, it's considered unethical to withhold it. Controlled trials then become hard to justify, which discourages the development of better forms of therapy.

Nonetheless, some question Wellcome's position. Although 260 patients is "an adequate number for this drug trial, it has more to do with hard cash than with altruism," says Dan William, a New York physician who devotes most of his practice to AIDS patients. "I'm almost certain that was the limiting factor." The company is, after all, paying the entire $5 million cost.

Even if AZT fails, says King, Wellcome is determined to gain something from this trial—namely, a method for testing the next AIDS drug, and a sense of which lab tests and symptoms truly reflect the course of the still poorly understood disease.

Some patients in the trial feel that this information is being gathered unfairly at their expense. "It's guinea pig city," says one. "They're rather arrogant. They know they've got you, because they're holding out this thread of a chance of life. They give you just enough capsules—oh, maybe a couple extra—to keep you going until your next appointment. You have to take the capsules every four hours, even during the night, and you're not supposed to take them within an hour of eating. That's the hardest part, planning your meals, because AIDS does strange things to your appetite. And then you realize you're going through all this agony and you might be bringing home sugar pills."

One of his nightmares is that he'll be dropped from the trial. He thinks certain illnesses could disqualify him, but he doesn't know which ones. "I had a real shock one week when I casually mentioned that I had taken aspirin," he says. "They practically went into orbit. They want you cold turkey on everything. I've taken some drugs to control other things, and I haven't told them. I don't tell them all my symptoms, either. This is life and death. The word is that once you're on the study they really don't want to throw you off, because they don't want to lose a patient, lose the data. But who wants to take a chance?"

The people who draw blood and ask questions at the hospital never tell him how he's doing, and he doesn't ask. "I assume all the blood is sent away, and they don't even know the results themselves, because it might bias them. And if they did know anything, I assume they wouldn't tell. But I'm having tests run, trying to monitor it on my own. I'd like to take the capsules to a lab and have them analyzed to see if they're placebos, but I haven't gotten far with that." If he learned he was getting a placebo—and he's convinced that he is—he wouldn't let on. "I'd probably keep going through the motions so as not to hurt my chances of ever getting the drug," he says. "I wish I were getting this drug. I really do."

He has no idea what will happen to him at the end of the trial, if he lives that long. If he's getting the drug, he assumes it will be withdrawn, at least until the results are analyzed. If he isn't, he's been assured he'll be on the list to get it if it works. "But God knows when they'll have the results. And time is such a factor in this disease."

Some researchers say this attitude is fairly common, and understandable, among patients who find that a placebo-controlled trial offers them their only chance to try a drug that might help them. Other scientists profess horror that a patient would break his word and do things to undermine the trial. Two doctors, both of whom conduct clinical trials with AIDS patients, commented on this patient's story. Dr. B also commented on Dr. A's remarks.

Doctor A: A patient like that doesn't belong in a clinical trial. Frankly, it sounds to me as if he has psychiatric problems.

Doctor B: That sounds like a doctor who shouldn't be running a clinical trial. *He* is the one with the psychiatric problem: he doesn't know what it's like to be ill.

Another patient with AIDS, who says he believes in the trial, is also taking other drugs secretly, simply because he thinks he needs them. And he, too—with the cooperation of his personal doctor—is concealing important symptoms from the researchers, for fear of being kicked out of the trial. A third patient likes being part of the experiment because he feels reassured by having his health monitored so closely, because he'll be among the first to get the drug if it proves to be effective, and because he likes the idea of helping to bring about something that may benefit others. The researchers discuss his test results with him; he doesn't think information is being withheld. If he takes an aspirin or a sleeping pill, he tells them, and they just record the information. He wouldn't consider taking prohibited drugs or having his capsules analyzed, or doing anything else that might ruin the trial. But, he says, he has a very early case of ARC, and, "according to the doctors, I'm the healthiest person on the protocol. Things might be different if I were deteriorating."

Many AIDS patients are apparently taking antiviral drugs on their own. Given these circumstances, is it even possible to conduct a placebo-controlled trial? King thinks eight out of ten patients are following the rule that bars other medications, mostly out of respect for the purpose of the trial. "I'm counting on the wisdom of these patients," he says. He's also counting on blood and urine tests to tell him who's cheating. Patients found to be taking drugs that interfere with the experiment will be thrown out, he says—"although I can't think of an occasion when we've thrown a patient off for this. In fact, we've stretched our imaginations to keep them on the study. I think sometimes our clinical investigators [the doctors running the trials at the medical centers] scare the hell out of patients" on this point. "It makes them comply," he says. But he's impressed by the ingenious forms that noncompliance can take: "We have two patients manifesting things we know to be traits of very sensitive responders to AZT. Yet one of them is supposed to be on placebo." He thinks the two have tried to improve their odds of getting AZT by swapping half their capsules.

King says that only rarely are patients dropped from the trial because they develop infections or other disorders. Patients who get sick, he says, are given whatever drugs they need in addition to AZT—unless their illness appears to be caused by AZT itself, or to require such "extremes of medical management" that they can no longer participate in the trial. He declines comment on a case reported by Barbara Starrett, a New York internist who has treated more than a hundred AIDS patients. "I had one patient who had just started on the study when he got cryptococcal meningitis and was thrown out," says Starrett. "There was concern because the medicine for meningitis is so strong. I had to Federal Express his medication back to the company. His father wrote them a letter, saying 'My son did his part, and now you won't let him continue.' It was really heartrending."

Starrett has other serious reservations about the trial: "It doesn't make sense to have half the patients getting placebos when you know they're just going to die, or get sicker. You know the natural course of this disease over six months. Double blind, control groups, and so on—it's all very academic. With AIDS, you don't need it. And I think they could get statistically significant information in less than six months. Another problem is that they want people on no other drugs, not even prophylaxis for pneumocystis pneumonia." Starrett and other doctors believe that certain powerful antibiotics do work, not against AIDS itself, but in warding off some of the devastating infections it brings. "For the placebo group, it's horrible, putting them on a study and telling them they can't take anything to prevent opportunistic infections," she says.

Such arguments aren't easily dismissed. More than half of the 22,000 AIDS cases diagnosed in the U.S. since 1981 have ended in death. The average life expectancy from the time of diagnosis is two years; those who come down with opportunistic infections like pneumocystis pneumonia may survive only six months. And many researchers now think that even before symptoms develop, the virus has already invaded the brain, where it may do irreversible damage.

Last May, at a public meeting in New York about AIDS, Mathilde Krim, a scientist who has taken up the cause of AIDS patients with a particular passion, described the AZT trial as "morally unacceptable." She cited the small number of patients, the use of placebos, Wellcome's refusal to release AZT for compassionate use, and the six-month treatment period, during which, she predicted, many of the controls would die. "AZT currently appears to be the most promising treatment," Krim says. "Ten thousand victims are being denied the drug that they and their doctors believe holds the most hope. It should be possible to resolve the need for scientific data with justice and compassion."

Krim, a Swiss-trained geneticist and associate research scientist at the St. Luke's–Roosevelt Hospital Center in New York, began studying AIDS in 1982. She and a colleague run a private foundation that recently awarded $1.6 million to other scientists working on the disease. In addition, she has served on several national advisory panels concerned with medical and scientific ethics. Krim suggests ways of testing AZT that get around the problem of leaving the control patients untreated. At the top of her list are the use of "historical controls"—the medical records of untreated patients of the past—as the control group, and the comparison of AZT to ribavirin, an antiviral drug whose effect on AIDS isn't known but whose toxicity is; she suggests "crossover" experiments that would let each group try both drugs.

She also believes that AZT should be supplied for compassionate use to patients who don't qualify for clinical trials and who have very little time left—those who have had pneumocystis pneumonia more than once, for instance, or who are showing signs of brain infection. If Burroughs Wellcome can't or won't make enough AZT, she thinks the federal government ought to let contracts out to other companies and supply it to patients without charge. "What about the guy who can expect to live six months?" she says. "If he's willing to take a chance, if he wants it so badly, why not give it to him? They'll say, 'It may be toxic, we've killed mice with AZT.' That's idiotic. We can kill mice with sugar and salt and mother's milk. We're too paternalistic, and in this case paternalism coincides with commercial interests."

Krim made her case again on July 1, before a hearing in Washington held by New York Democrat Ted Weiss's House subcommittee on intergovernmental relations and human resources. "Do we not owe all those who are dying a small measure of hope, if we can provide it, and the dignity they so want, to fight to the end?" she asked. Three other witnesses supported her: two AIDS patients and a Cleveland physician, who criticized the lack of government funding for AIDS trials in Ohio, which has made it impossible for most of his patients to get experimental drugs. But other witnesses—including researchers and representatives of drug companies and federal health agencies—differed. Massachusetts General Hospital physician Martin Hirsch said, "Our goal must not be to have everyone on some drug of uncertain value, but to have every patient in a clinical trial from which useful information may result."

"Dr. Krim has a very strong, compelling argument," says King. "I've heard it used in the past by people who had decided for whatever reason that an agent was effective. If you accept her premise that this agent is effective, then you have to agree with her. I don't accept her premise. Perhaps she has come away from that *Lancet* paper, as many have, with wishful thinking. And if another agent had been available to test AZT against, neither the FDA nor the institutional review boards [the medical-center groups that must approve research involving human subjects] would've allowed placebos. I think Dr. Krim is so desperate for an agent to be effective that she's not thinking too clearly about it."

Krim herself acknowledges that she isn't an expert in the design of clinical trials, and indeed many researchers more experienced than she in this area say her suggestions just wouldn't work. It's true that placebos are considered ethically unacceptable once an effective, well studied drug is available for use as a basis for comparison. But there's no such drug for AIDS. In this situation, says John C. Bailar III, a physician and medical statistician who teaches at the Harvard School of Public Health, a control group that receives supportive therapy when needed—but not the test drug—"is mandatory." AZT doesn't appear to exert what he calls a "wham-bang effect: you don't see patients rising from their death beds." Without an untreated group, it would be too easy—particularly in a disease with such a variable course—to miss less dramatic, though still important, effects. Historical controls are out of the question, Bailar says, because new patients differ from old ones in two key ways: the disease tends to get diagnosed earlier nowadays, and, as doctors gain experience treating the various infections and cancers, the course of the disease, and even life expectancy, may be changing.

Comparing AZT to another drug instead of a placebo could be not only confusing but dangerous, according to Broder. Suppose, he suggests, that researchers unwittingly chose as a basis for comparison a drug that actually made patients worse. Then even ineffective test drugs would look good. This could confound trials for years to come. Nonetheless, Broder says of Krim's opinions, "I respect that view very much. But declaring a drug to be effective before you know it to be effective and safe won't help anybody."

Levine agrees that placebo-controlled trials are the most efficient means of testing new drugs, but says, "There are limits to what we do in the name of efficiency. To justify the use of placebos, or of any controlled trial—and I think there's pretty near consensus on this—you must have no reason to believe there's any difference between the two things you're testing." When the early evidence in favor of a drug is strong, he says, controlled trials are unwarranted. In the case of AZT, the first trial didn't provide enough evidence, so controls are needed. Placebo controls would be acceptable with patients who have ARC, he told Weiss's subcommittee, but "almost impossible" to justify in patients with full-blown AIDS. Because the prognosis is so bad, it would be ethically preferable to treat them.

William is also ambivalent. "I hate it and I love it," he says of the AZT trial. "I hate it because it's very unfair to all the people who are waiting for answers, because the inclusion criteria are so narrow, because they have patients getting up at four o'clock every morning for months and months to take placebos, and because they're drawing blood and examining and testing them all the time.

"I love it because narrow inclusion criteria and a long follow-up are the best way to get answers fast. It's a clean study"—statistically clean, in that it should prove beyond a doubt whether or not AZT works—"but it's mean."

Ronald Grossman, another New York doctor who treats many AIDS patients, takes a different view: he wants experimental drugs for his patients, and thinks such drugs should be available on a compassionate basis for those who can't get into trials. And the trials themselves ought to be conducted without placebos, he says; one alternative would be to treat all the patients, but with different doses of the same drug, and compare those results. But this approach would take longer, he acknowledges, and perhaps yield fuzzier data. "It's a terrible dilemma," he says. "Dare we sacrifice scientific methods, or dare we let thousands die in the lag period, for the so-called greater good?" He favors choosing as controls those patients who don't want drug treatment. They do exist, he says, though of course in small numbers. This summer, Grossman and Krim will meet with Otis Bowen, secretary of the Department of Health and Human Services, to urge more government spending to make new AIDS drugs available.

Some scientists point to the past year's experience with a drug called suramin as an omen about what can go wrong with a treatment that starts out looking right. The drug had been in use for many years as a treatment for several parasitic diseases, when Broder and his colleagues tested it for six weeks in ten AIDS patients; their results aroused a great deal of hope and enthusiasm, because suramin stopped the AIDS virus from replicating in several of the patients.

"Here was the first hint of a possibility on the horizon of an antiviral drug to treat this dreaded disease," says Bruce Cheson, who coordinated a series of suramin studies sponsored by the NCI. "We of course were flooded with requests from patients, their relatives, and institutions, asking us to release the drug on a compassionate plea basis. We took a fairly strong position." Because of side effects—rashes, fevers, and changes in liver function—and uncertainties about dosage, Cheson says, the NCI concluded that making suramin widely available to doctors "wasn't a safe thing to do." Instead, it set up studies at six hospitals for only about a hundred patients in all.

"Suramin had substantial antiviral activity," says Cheson. "But it produced no immunological improvement, and clinical responses were uncommon. And it didn't cross the blood-brain barrier." Most important, more than a quarter of the patients who took it developed adrenal insufficiency, a potentially serious and completely unanticipated side effect. Since some of its symptoms mimic those of AIDS itself, the adrenal disorder might not have been recognized had the drug been widely distributed instead of being tested at academic centers that routinely ran lab tests to gauge adrenal function. Suramin may have even killed a few patients, according to Cheson, by damaging their livers. "Suramin taught us to limit compassionate use," he says. "We need to take a firm stand on this, to avoid harming people."

Another drug, HPA-23—the one that Rock Hudson went to
Paris for—has been in use for several years, but doctors still don't
know whether it works. And most researchers agree that the confusion is due to the lack of controlled trials of the drug.

Dr. Anthony Fauci, the director of the National Institute of
Allergy and Infectious Diseases, which sponsors a great deal of
the AIDS research in the U.S., is incensed by ideas like Mathilde
Krim's, particularly when they come from scientists who, like
Krim, work in the laboratory and don't treat patients. "I spend
most of my life treating AIDS patients," he says, his voice rising
to a level between talking and shouting, and staying there for
about forty minutes. The very idea that an ethical problem might
arise from the use of untreated controls seems to strike him as ab-
surd. "Untreated? Untreated with what? *There is no treatment, no
proved drug*. Do you think there's some kind of conspiracy among
researchers to use placebos and let the patients die?" AZT has received more publicity than it deserves, he says. Fauci insists that
except for "miracle drugs," which he asserts AZT is definitely
not, there's no alternative to a placebo-controlled trial. Releasing
the drug for widespread use now would make it virtually impossible to study, he says. "It would be an absolute tragedy if five years
from now, because of being compassionate, with good intentions,
we had no idea what worked and what didn't. Because by 1991,
there will be 271,000 people with AIDS in this country alone.
Yes, we have to have compassion for the individual patient, but
we also have a responsibility to the larger group."

But what about compassionate use restricted to patients with
the very worst outlook, those with signs of brain infection, for instance, or those who fit into some narrowly defined group, as do
the patients in the current trial? "What if there's a shortage of the
drug?" asks Fauci. What if there isn't? "What if there's a chance
that the drug will kill them off just before another drug is proved
effective?" asks Fauci. What if they want to take that chance? "I
don't see how it could be done," he says. The rules would be impossible to enforce. "Those things break down." But finally he
says, "If it didn't interfere with the ability to answer the
question"—meaning the question of whether the drug is
effective—"I wouldn't object."

With AIDS victims dying at the rate of about 175 a week in
the U.S., it's hard to argue with a scientific approach that's so

widely regarded as the fastest way to figure out whether AZT works, and that may help researchers evaluate other drugs more quickly. If AZT proves effective, it will probably never be necessary to do another placebo-controlled trial again, because AZT will become the standard that other drugs will have to measure up to. But if the results are equivocal, the end of the current test may just mean the beginning of more tests. And yet, if such experiments fail to provide the needed information, it may become harder and harder to justify them to patients. At the same time, if it's possible to carry out rigorous, tightly controlled trials, it should be possible to let drugs out on a limited, tightly controlled, compassionate basis, for patients who are willing to take a chance and whose time is short. Research can serve the individual and society; compassion and responsibility aren't mutually exclusive. In the words of a 33-year-old AIDS victim, "All I have to cling to is hope. And hope comes in the form of new drugs."

EDITOR'S NOTE: In October 1986 the New York *Times* announced that the test group for AZT had been broadened to include 7,000 patients.

AIDS AND LAWYERS[8]

There were encouraging reports last month that scientists are making great progress in developing a vaccine against AIDS. Unfortunately, under present legal conditions, even if such a vaccine were available tomorrow, no one would produce it.

Suppose the research and development department at the Mammoth Drug Company *does* come up with an AIDS vaccine. The scientists test it on monkeys and rats, and it works. The microbiologists say it's a sure bet to work on humans too. What next? To start with, a lengthy review of the record by the Food and Drug Administration. Then tightly supervised human testing in limited populations. Federal law is clear: drugs are not allowed on the market until they are proven not merely "safe," but

[8]Reprint of an article by Peter Huber, Washington attorney. Reprinted by permission from *New Republic*, 194:14–15. My. 5, '86. Copyright © 1986 by *New Republic*.

"effective" as well. The same testing is required whether the drug treats AIDS or acne. The earliest conceivable FDA approval is two years down the line.

And probably a lot longer. There's a good chance the new vaccine—like many of the old ones used against other diseases— will be a living (but weakened) virus. This crippled AIDS virus almost certainly will have been developed by genetic engineering. And today's regulators are deeply nervous about gene-altered organisms. Any kind of testing outside a triply secure lab will require interminable advance review. The Agriculture Department recently prompted a front-page controversy after it cut some corners in approving a gene-modified vaccine for a pseudo-rabies that is deadly to swine. Approving a genetically altered bug that looks a lot like the AIDS virus will lead to a much bigger fuss.

But maybe Washington would throw out the rule book for something as politically urgent as AIDS. Assume an AIDS vaccine could get prompt blessing. Next step: manufacture. But most vaccines have side effects of some type or another. Remember swine flu? The vaccine against the disease turned out to cause Guillain-Barre syndrome in some who received it. Whooping cough? The pertussis vaccine occasionally causes death or serious brain damage. Sabin polio vaccine? Responsible for an occasional case of polio. The benefit of taking all these vaccines far outweighs the tiny risk of side effects. But for those very few who lose the gamble, the temptation to sue is overwhelming.

Of course, the FDA testing might uncover the AIDS-vaccine side effects before Mammoth goes to market. But then again, it might not. FDA tests will be carried to the point where everyone is sure that the vaccine cures more disease than it causes. But that's about all that a limited test of 2,000 persons can ever tell you. There's no way the FDA can nail down the one-in-a-million human side effect without actually vaccinating a million people. Even if the FDA discovers a side effect, this doesn't mean that the vaccine won't—or shouldn't—be produced. It just means that manufacturers will be able to warn people of the possible side effect before they take the vaccine, which may provide some legal protection. But there can be no warning against side effects that are unknown.

And what are the occasional side effects of the AIDS vaccine likely to be if they do materialize after mass inoculations? Impossible to say. But there's a fair chance that for the tiniest fraction of those vaccinated the side effect will be AIDS itself, or something equally horrible. Hearing this, the general counsel at Mammoth Drug may have a stroke. He's been spending a lot of time in court recently, defending vaccine lawsuits, and without much success. He knows, for example, that a polio victim in Kansas successfully sued American Cyanamid for ten million dollars in 1984. The vaccine was fine, made just as the FDA requires. But one unlucky recipient suffered the side effects that neither the FDA nor Mammoth knows how to eliminate, and a jury was feeling generous. It happens. In the case of vaccines, it happens often.

Even if the risks from the vaccine are very small—much smaller than the risks from AIDS itself—the financial stakes are huge. Weird and unexpected things happen in drug litigation. Look what happened with a swine flu vaccine. All those who contracted Guillain-Barre syndrome within two months of receiving the vaccine were compensated for their illnesses, even though as many as half of the cases were not caused by the vaccine.

Suppose the AIDS vaccine is perfectly safe for most people, but causes allergic reactions in those who have already been exposed to AIDS. Mammoth could end up paying dearly, even if it warns everyone of the risk. Somewhere, somehow, the wrong person will still get vaccinated. Or even more likely, the *right* person will be vaccinated: someone for whom the one-in-a-million side effect is clearly a risk worth taking (just as taking the polio vaccine is well worth the infinitesimal risk today). But then the side effect will strike, and the victim will claim he wasn't sufficiently warned. Faced with a sympathetic victim, a jury can be adept at rereading the fine print of a warning and finding it inadequate. If the new AIDS vaccine gets out there on the market, scratched into the arms of millions of people, and it turns out to have *any* side effects to speak of, Mammoth could go under.

Mammoth's general counsel does not plan to preside over the bankruptcy-court dismantling of his corporate empire. Remember Johns-Manville and asbestos? A. H. Robbins and the Dalkon Shield? Those firms may indeed have been negligent, but that's small comfort to the Mammoth general counsel. He will remind the Mammoth board of directors that negligence is always easier to find in hindsight. No doubt he will also remind them that Wyeth Laboratories halted manufacture of the whooping cough vaccine in 1984, citing dramatic increases in insurance and litigation costs. Dozens of other companies have left the vaccine market in the last 15 years for similar reasons.

The lawsuits that are driving companies out of the vaccine business generally don't even allege negligence in manufacture. They usually turn on arguments about how the warning on the package was phrased, or on fancy theories of liability without fault. Any theory will do, if it might get a case to the jury. Knowing this, nervous companies settle—and then get out of the vaccine business.

Our Mammoth Drug Company can't buy comprehensive insurance for any vaccine marketing, and neither can anyone else. Why not? The general counsel at Colossal Insurance doesn't care for bankruptcy any more than her brother at Mammoth. Selfish, but a very real fact of today's marketplace. This fact was made clear ten years ago, during the swine flu scare. Congress rushed through some emergency legislation, assuming responsibility for the vaccine's side effects (which were pinned down well after the program got under way). The pharmaceutical companies were required to sell the vaccine at cost, realizing not a penny of profit. The Justice Department spent the next ten years dealing with millions in liability claims. They're still digging out.

Of course, Congress might well get around to raising the legislative umbrella over the new AIDS vaccine too. There's already a bill before the California legislature designed to guarantee the purchase of an AIDS vaccine, and protect its manufacturer from liability. But it's only a bill, and only in one state. And if Mammoth has to rely on this, or on the federal swine flu model, the profit in its AIDS vaccine will be unimpressive.

So what exactly does Mammoth have to gain from pushing its AIDS research? The corporate research scientists are terribly excited, of course—there's probably a Nobel Prize waiting out there. The PR people would love to draft the new ads for the evening news: "Mammoth Drug: People to the Aid of People." And there might be some money to be made on the vaccine in Europe and Canada. The Rock Hudsons of the world could undoubtedly pay a premium to get the vaccine overseas. All of this might be enough to keep a modest amount of research going. But research microbiologists come very expensive these days—not to mention the equipment and laboratories they need. Testing to satisfy the

FDA is expensive too. Even if there are still potential profits, a few lawsuits could swallow them all. But all in all, these are slim pickings. Better for Mammoth to send most of the R&D boys back to the mass-market nasal sprays.

III. CONTROVERSIES AND ETHICAL ISSUES

EDITOR'S INTRODUCTION

Since AIDS was first diagnosed, efforts to cope with the disease have been hampered by fear, prejudice, and confusion in the public mind. Because a large percentage of those affected have been homosexuals, hostility rather than compassion has been directed at the victims. A number of church leaders have openly expressed satisfaction that these individuals' lives have been taken by divine justice, and "gay bashing"—from proliferating AIDS jokes to physical assaults—has been widespread. In certain cases these AIDS victims have been sacked from their jobs, or evicted from their dwellings, becoming pariahs. With a flow of information in the media, a more rational response to AIDS has been evolving, but controversies of various kinds remain.

The first article in this section, an editorial in the *Nation,* charges that the Reagan administration's response to AIDS has been tardy and half-hearted, and that an "atmosphere of extreme social squeamishness and a medieval moralism" have impeded an enlightened response to this public health issue. Another editorial, in the *New Republic,* blames the public's fear over how AIDS can be caught on the misinformation of media coverage and ambiguous official assurances that merely raise alarm. In his article in *Newsweek,* Jonathan Alter defends media coverage as being increasingly responsible, while conceding that the press has not reported clearly on the specifics of AIDS (i.e., its transmission through anal sex) out of fear of offending the public's sensibilities. All of these articles touch on the issue of the politics of AIDS, on the conflict between a public health crisis and a disinclination to confront it candidly because its victims often belong to an unpopular minority group.

Jerry Adler's article "The AIDS Conflict," from *Newsweek,* addresses the panic over AIDS that has led to boycotts of schools when a child having AIDS was admitted to classes with other children, and to the demand by some that all AIDS victims should be quarantined. Another article, in *Fortune* magazine, raises the issue of discrimination by insurance companies, who have developed methods of assessing risks through "lifestyle clues" (single males, for example, in large cities). The subject of the two following articles is discrimination in the workplace. An article in the *Economist* notes the Justice Department's ruling that the 1973 federal law prohibiting job discrimination against the handicapped applies to those who have AIDS but not to those who are thought to have been exposed to AIDS yet have not come down with the disease. The Attorney General's opinion, the article points out, would make "more than a million not-yet-sick people unemployable." In a related article in *Newsweek*, Matt Clark examines the illogicality of the ruling further. As Clark indicates, the ruling purports to protect other workers from contagion—despite doctors' repeated assurances that the disease cannot be spread through casual contact. If the federal government establishes an illogical guideline, how can companies in the private sector be expected to respond to the issue of discrimination clear-sightedly?

A SOCIAL DISEASE[1]

Diseases have social as well as biological histories, and it is impossible to consider any affliction independent of the complex cultural syndrome in which it thrives. Cancer is not just a matter of oncogenes and mutagens but a consequence of political decisions, economic practices, technological developments and personal habits. Toxic shock syndrome was identified, publicized, analyzed and eventually made curable in large part because of the feminist movement's aggressive interest in women's health and sexual issues. Approaches to mental illness, alcoholism and severe physical handicaps demonstrate the inseparability of policy and therapy.

AIDS is a social disease in every sense of the phrase. It is transmitted by intimate contact, but more than that, it is encountered in terms of social paranoia, political prejudice and cultural ignorance. AIDS is endemic in equatorial Africa, where it takes its toll

---

[1] Reprint of *Nation* editorial. Reprinted by permission from *The Nation*, 241:195–6. S. 14, '85. Copyright © 1985 by *The Nation*.

in millions, without regard to gender, sexual preference or drug dependence. But Americans care little for foreign victims of deadly agents, even when those are international in scope of provenance. We say that 50,000 died in Vietnam without mentioning the dead millions who were not born in the U.S.A. The media finds comfort in reporting that few or no Americans were aboard a plane that plunged into a distant peak, though the craft was made in Seattle. And who considers the people slaughtered in a far-off jungle, even though the impetus and the wherewithal for the massacre came from the heart of America?

At the start, then, AIDS patients all over the world are affected not only by a deadly retrovirus but by the racial, national and geographical pattern of the epidemic. In the United States, the 12,000 people who have thus far contracted the disease have also been beset by an atmosphere of extreme social squeamishness and a medieval moralism that is proving as lethal as their symptoms.

In a kind of public health vigilantism, discrimination against AIDS victims is spreading, and opportunities for institutional gay-bashing abound. A school board in Queens, New York, defies the superintendent's call to admit carefully screened children who have the disease. The Army announces that it will give all new enlistees a test, now administered to blood donors, which determines the presence of an AIDS antibody, not the disease itself. The screening seems obviously designed to keep homosexuals out of the Army because of their sexuality and not because of any health hazard. Some insurance companies are hiring private investigators to ascertain if applicants are homosexual. That practice could result in the denial of coverage to millions of non-afflicted gay men solely because they are in a high-risk group. And in New York City, with about one-third of all U.S. cases, the government does little to help victims, disseminate health information or fund services that could ease the crisis. Mayor Koch, now up for reelection, defies all medical advice and urges that children with AIDS be barred from school and thus made pariahs.

Because a majority of the victims are homosexual or are otherwise stigmatized by society, the authorities who control medical funds have been unwilling to finance the comprehensive campaigns required to develop preventive and therapeutic regimens. It simply is not true, as Health and Human Services Secretary

Margaret Heckler asserted this summer, that the government is spending all the money that can be usefully absorbed by researchers. Virtually every scientist and social worker fighting AIDS believes that there is a direct correlation between spending money and saving lives, that it is technically possible to speed up the process of developing a vaccine to prevent the disease and producing antiviral methods to control it.

Only one of many tragic ironies of the AIDS epidemic is that its victims, and those who are at greatest risk of infection, have to wait for its spread to more celebrated groups before much progress will be made. Rock Hudson's case may well generate enough publicity to save thousands of others; Heckler threw a few more millions into the project after Hudson's diagnosis was made public. Now the news media has discovered that heterosexuals, too, are worried about contracting AIDS. In other words, it's time to get serious.

Somehow death and disease don't seem as dreadful when they befall other people—especially social groups that may conveniently be blamed for their own misery. Even starvation remains abstract until it affects people who count in the world, as *The New York Times* confirmed recently in a headline of classic snobbery: "Middle Class in Ethiopia Begins to Feel the Pinch of Famine." It's too bad that a businessman must go hungry or a movie star get sick before the world is moved to action.

AFRAIDS[2]

In 1983, the latest year for which statistics are available, 130 people, 55 of them students, died in school bus accidents. In that same year, as in all other years to date, zero students were diagnosed with AIDS infections incurred at school. If you were to stand up at your local school board meeting and demand that school buses be banned on the grounds that "any risk, however small, is too great when children are involved," you would not be

[2]Reprint of *New Republic* editorial. Reprinted by permission from the *New Republic*, 193:7–8. O. 14, '85. Copyright © 1985 by *New Republic*.

treated seriously. Yet that is precisely the logic that is carrying the day in many school districts about letting children with AIDS into the classroom.

It is true that not everything is known about AIDS, and it is understandable that parents wish to take no chances where the welfare of their children is concerned. But contrary to what they have been led to believe by many in the media, the transmission of AIDS is far from an utter mystery. As conservatives often point out in other contexts, the search for a perfectly risk-free environment is not only futile, but it also creates costs of its own. In the case of AIDS, the cost is partly a moral one.

The AIDS issue has now spawned a second epidemic—a wave of hysteria whose symptoms include ostracism, discrimination, and violence. As with other communicable maladies, we'll give this hysteria a name: Acute Fear Regarding AIDS or, more simply, AFRAIDS. Surveys indicate that whereas AIDS has thus far struck only a small fraction of the population, AFRAIDS has already infected well over a hundred million people. According to a recent *New York Times*/CBS poll, 47 percent of Americans believe it is possible to catch AIDS from a shared drinking glass, 28 percent implicate contaminated toilet seats, and 12 percent consider themselves endangered by a shared office environment or even a carrier's touch. Meanwhile, a *Washington Post* survey found that 34 percent of those polled considered it unsafe to "associate" with an AIDS victim—even when no physical contact was involved—and an additional 22 percent were uncertain.

Thanks to such misconceptions, many unlucky AIDS casualties, already laboring under a death sentence, are victimized a second time—thrown out of jobs, apartments, and schools, harassed and discharged by the military, and rejected by roommates, friends, and family. Worse, patients have been barred from hospitals, denied ambulance services, and refused mouth-to-mouth resuscitation. Organizations and families offering refuge to patients have been greeted with bomb warnings, death threats, vandalism, and assault.

The worst form of the AFRAIDS contagion is transmission of the disease from parents to children. In Queens, fear of an AIDS-afflicted second-grader triggered a boycott in two school districts that kept over a quarter of the area's 47,000 elementary and junior high school students at home on the first day of classes. The September 23 *Newsweek* featured a sickening cover photograph of children carrying placards against other children ("NO AIDS CHILDREN IN DISTRICT 27"). Thirteen-year-old Ryan White, banned from school in Indiana, observed pointedly about this state of affairs, "It stinks."

Since August authorities at the Federal Centers of Disease Control have been trying to arrest the spread of misinformation and panic. In a recent report, the center concluded that "casual person-to-person contact, as among schoolchildren, appears to pose no risk." Again, in a September 13 interview in *The New York Times,* Dr. Martha Rogers, an AIDS epidemiologist at the CDC, assured the public that "we obviously believe the evidence thus far indicates that transmission by casual contact will never occur." Unfortunately, these efforts to alleviate panic have inadvertently backfired: decisive judgments such as "never" and "no risk" have been overshadowed in the public mind by caveats such as "appears," "believe," "thus far," and "indicates." Intended simply as gestures of obeisance to scientific protocol, these formal qualifications have been widely misinterpreted as confessions of general ignorance on the part of the medical profession.

Naturally, this atmosphere of uncertainty has encouraged the casual transmission of AFRAIDS. In July the cover of *Life* magazine alerted readers, "NOW NO ONE IS SAFE FROM AIDS." The word "AIDS," plastered in thick, blood-red letters, covered an area three inches tall and ten inches wide. Inside, the ostensible cause for alarm proved considerably thinner. What the article actually substantiated was that no one is safe from AIDS who has sex with a carrier or receives a contaminated blood transfusion.

Rupert Murdoch's *New York Post* has been at the forefront of the misinformation campaign. On September 12, the *Post*'s front page screamed, "SCHOOL COOK DIES OF AIDS." As if the hint of likely contamination weren't clear enough, the next day's cover followed with "Top doc's warning to schools: KEEP AIDS KIDS OUT." "Top doc" turned out to be Ronald Rosenblatt, a Queens internist with neither firsthand nor, apparently, thirdhand knowledge of reliable AIDS research.

The best evidence that AIDS can't be transmitted through casual contact is that not one of the family members of the 13,000 presently known AIDS victims (except for sexual partners and children infected in the womb) has developed AIDS symptoms, and none who has been tested is carrying the virus. As the CDC's Rogers observes, if you can't catch the bug by years of hugging, kissing, touching, and sharing food, utensils, and bathrooms with a carrier, chances are virtually nonexistent that you'll contract it just from sharing a classroom or an office. The AIDS virus has been isolated in saliva, tears, and urine. However, Rogers reports, "not one case of transmission from these fluids has ever been documented."

Skeptics raise two points most frequently in the face of this evidence. First, they note that the source of every AIDS victim's virus is not known. Specifically, ten percent of juvenile cases and six percent of adult cases remain unaccounted for. However, these leftover cases reflect procedural difficulties more than substantive doubts. Many juvenile cases cannot be formally closed simply because the mother, suspected of having passed the virus during pregnancy, is deceased or otherwise inaccessible. As for the adults, their cases will stay open as long as their lips remain sealed. The suspected routes—prostitute contact and homosexual activity—are not the sorts of hobbies a family man wants to reveal to his wife and children. In a recent study, a third of the unclassified adult male victims interviewed confessed to prostitute contact, and researchers hope and expect that further admissions will be forthcoming.

Second, skeptics point out that the incubation period of AIDS is several years. Only recently has there been a significant number of AIDS victims. Who is to say they aren't transmitting the disease in ways that won't become tragically apparent until years from now? In fact, the average time between infection and diagnosis of AIDS is one year for children, two for adults. AIDS has been under study for seven years, and yet not a single case of casual transmission has surfaced so far. What's more, among the 300 family members of AIDS victims who have had blood tests, none has shown the presence of the virus.

AIDS, like other infectious diseases, is transmittable after infection, and not just when the symptoms appear. The people developing AIDS now have been carriers for a long time. If the disease were transmittable in ways other than those that already have been established, this would show up now, not several years from now.

Whether with reckless opportunism or with the best of intentions, many publications—and even some physicians—have underscored routine uncertainties and voiced answerable doubts, falsely portraying this as the standpoint of "caution." The ironic result is the present epidemic explosion of AFRAIDS. Much of the public is now hopelessly confused, skeptical even to the point of questioning the sincerity of medical authorities. Dazed by the flurry of information and misinformation, lay people have simply resigned from the debate, concluding that the doctors don't have satisfactory answers. They await the day when medicine comes forth and declares unequivocally, in the words of President Reagan, "This we know for a fact, that it is safe." But this declaration is not likely to issue from the scrupulously cautious scientific community in this decade, perhaps not even in this century.

The question is, what do we do in the meantime? There is always—on a theoretical level—a risk that the AIDS kid at your local elementary school will engage your seven-year-old son in a fistfight, that both will bleed profusely, and that somehow the dastardly virus will worm its way across. There's even a hypothetical possibility that your child will catch the ailment just by drinking from the same water fountain or sitting in the same classroom. All logic and experience belies these fears, but they cannot be dismissed with absolute certainty. To some parents, landlords, and employers, this doesn't matter: a theoretical risk seems reason enough to exclude the infected individual from public life. Isn't that the counsel of caution? Isn't that the "safe" option?

Unfortunately, there is no safe option. Barring a child from school or excluding an adult from shelter and employment is not cost-free. It involves the expulsion not simply of a virus but of a human being. That must count for something. As a palpable cruelty, it seems a lot to ask for the sake of dispelling the darkest fantasies of the imagination.

SINS OF OMISSION[3]

If AIDS didn't exist, yellow journalism might have invented it. The story has every ingredient: sex, drugs, death and panic.

[3]Reprint of an article by Jonathan Alter, *Newsweek* staffwriter. Reprinted by permission from *Newsweek*, 106:25. S. 23, '85. Copyright © 1985 by *Newsweek*.

But except for the *New York Post* (TRAGIC FACES OF CAGED AIDS TOTS) and the supermarket tabloids (ROCK HUDSON'S LAST PLEA: LINDA, FORGIVE ME), the press has in general acted responsibly. (*Life* magazine— NOW NO ONE IS SAFE FROM AIDS —may have crossed the line, but not by much.) As the incidence of the disease has spread beyond New York and San Francisco, news organizations in other parts of the country have increased and improved their coverage—in some cases, even assigning top reporters full time to the story.

Even so, AIDS has proved an extraordinarily complex story to cover. One difficulty is that both print and electronic media are accustomed to certainty—a conviction that somewhere they can find the truth and report it. "We don't know" is an unsatisfactory closing line, even if it is sometimes the one most appropriate to this perplexing public-health threat. Given the linkage of AIDS with homosexuality, the disease also presents journalists with a highly charged social issue—and one that raises questions of taste. The result has been a series of sins of omission, some of which can lead to misinformation.

Perhaps the most common problem is a squeamish lack of specificity. Until quite recently, almost every television news program and large numbers of newspapers have observed an informal taboo. The disease is often said to be transmitted by "intimate sexual contact" or "exchange of bodily fluids." While much remains unknown about how the AIDS virus spreads, no description is really complete without reference to breakage of the rectal lining through anal sex. That is probably how the vast majority of the cases have been transmitted so far—a fact that underlines the remoteness of the AIDS risk from most people's experience. "Perhaps I need to be more specific," concedes Rosalind Jackler, the medical writer for *The Houston Post.* "I never really thought about it until now."

Bathhouses: Similarly, nowadays reporters rarely point out the correlation between AIDS and extreme promiscuity (dozens or even hundreds of sex partners). And few newspapers have called editorially for the closure of the remaining gay bathhouses, implicitly accepting the dubious argument of some gay activists that the issue is more one of civil liberties than health. With few exceptions—most notably an article in the Sept. 8 *Washington Post* by neurologist Richard Restak—the press has given little credence to those who believe that short of harder medical information it may eventually be necessary to separate victims from the rest of society.

The press on occasion seems almost oversolicitous of high-risk groups: "Because most reporters don't have much of an understanding of the gay community, they often get very nervous and don't want to offend," says Rodger Streitmatter, director of the print-journalism program at American University. And offense is easily given. *San Francisco Chronicle* reporter Randy Shilts, the first openly gay reporter to be assigned to cover exclusively gay issues, says that when he pointed out the hazards of bath-houses he was repeatedly denounced as a "gay Uncle Tom."

The sensitivity of gays is understandable, especially given the occasional gay-bashing in the press. In May 1983, for instance, syndicated columnist Patrick Buchanan, now director of communications at the White House, wrote that "[homosexuals] have declared war upon nature, and now nature is exacting an awful retribution." And the suggestion that casual contact can spread the disease ("He Chopped Green Beans & Roast Beef," read one subheadline of a *New York Post* story about an AIDS victim who was a public-school cook) has contributed to both hysteria and homophobia. In their presentation, however, many news organizations are trying to dispel rumor-induced panic. Many newspapers and magazines have run dry question-and-answer stories to counter unfounded public fears. And ABC's *20/20* is currently planning a segment in which Barbara Walters will hold a toddler with AIDS in order to help show that the child poses no threat.

Estimates: Another problem of the coverage has less to do with the press than with the "experts": because so little is known about AIDS, they often express differing views of the disease. On the *CBS Morning News* last week, for example, a University of California doctor said that heterosexual men rarely contracted AIDS from women; moments later, a Harvard doctor said that was incorrect. *The Washington Post* reported that 600,000 to 1.2 million might be infected, while *The Atlanta Constitution* put the number infected at 2 million and reported that as many as a third may get AIDS or some of its debilitating symptoms. While these stories drew a distinction between those with AIDS, which is invariably fatal, and those carrying the virus, who may not even get sick, the difference is frequently blurred. But when the distinction is drawn, the implication of some of the stories' infection statistics is huge fatality totals—as many Americans as died in World War

II. The possibility of widespread death has not often been broached publicly—perhaps because the press doesn't want to appear alarmist.

In New York, where more than 2,000 people have already died from AIDS, a careful reading of the *Times*'s obituary page is required for a full understanding of the impact of the disease. Not too many years ago, bereaved families considered the word "cancer" taboo in obits. Now cancer—sometimes the specific cause of death (along with pneumonia) after the immune system has been destroyed—is itself frequently used as a euphemism for AIDS. Like the others, this euphemism probably will disappear as the press and public learn to deal with a disease that both find terrifying—and difficult to comprehend.

THE AIDS CONFLICT[4]

Let us try to imagine a rational, humane approach towards AIDS. We will begin with two cases. One, which was much in the news last week, is that of a seven-year-old girl who was diagnosed as having AIDS three years ago and is still infectious, although well enough to attend school. New York City school officials, weighing the minuscule risk that she might go berserk in the lunchroom and bite another pupil, allowed her to begin second grade last week—a decision that touched off a lawsuit and an angry boycott involving as many as 18,000 children. The other concerns a homosexual man in Alameda County, Calif., who came down with the disease about the same time, and since then has been treated several times at the county public-health clinic for gonorrhea. He has sexual relations with three to five different men each week, without telling them of his condition. Dr. Robert Benjamin of the county Bureau of Communicable Diseases calls him "a sociopath," although he apparently is breaking no laws.

The only thing these cases have in common is that the awful medical complications of AIDS have been at least temporarily checked—with the result, ironically, that the ethical complica-

⁴Reprint of an article by Jerry Adler, *Newsweek* staffwriter. Reprinted by permission from *Newsweek*, 106:18–24. S. 23, '85. Copyright ©1985 by *Newsweek*.

tions have become even more vexing. The challenge is for us to fashion an approach that will do justice to both the extremes of innocence and depravity—and escape the one epidemic against which not even clean living is proof, an epidemic of fear. It won't be easy. Most doctors, let alone the public, had never heard of AIDS four or five years ago. Today information and misinformation about the disease are everywhere, and society is only now beginning to ask questions that may take the rest of this decade or longer to answer.

The smell of fear is already abroad; it is the smell of the insecticide with which a north-side Atlanta man was dousing his backyard one recent afternoon, defending against mosquitoes who might have just taken a nip out of one of the guests at his gay neighbor's barbecue. The sound of fear is echoing through the Hollywood hills—the hollow smack of lips on air as acquaintances duck the show-business kiss of greeting. To see the sight of fear, you'd have to be invited up to the bedroom of Jon-Henri Damski, columnist for Chicago's GayLife newspaper, where a poster describing sexual activities which do *not* spread AIDS hangs in a conspicuous spot above his bed.

The fear has brought us to the brink of major changes in our society, the result, as is so often the case, of technology outpacing wisdom. The development of a test to indicate whether a person has been exposed to the AIDS virus has made the nation's blood supply almost entirely safe again. But it also may enable health authorities, insurance companies and employers to identify individuals who are at risk of developing the disease, although they may appear perfectly healthy now and may never get sick. No one knows how many people that might be—but the U.S. Centers for Disease Control, which had been citing a range of 500,000 to 1 million, has quietly begun referring to an upper limit of 2 million. For the first time, talk of a quarantine, previously confined to a handful of gay-baiting crackpots, has begun appearing in such high-minded forums as *The Washington Post*—while William Curran, professor of legal medicine at Harvard Medical School, told *Newsweek* that he is preparing standby regulations for cities to apply in confining AIDS patients who willfully persist in giving the disease to others.

And these changes will occur against a background of sheer ignorance that no amount of scientific information seems capable of dispelling. The leading researchers who have studied AIDS are unanimous in saying that it is known to be transmitted in only two ways: by sexual contact, especially among homosexual men, or by exposure to infected blood. Virtually every public mention of the disease underscores this point, yet a *New York Times*/CBS News poll last week found that nearly half the population thought they could catch AIDS by sharing a glass with a patient. The fact that AIDS has been transmitted by transfusions of infected blood has led a number of people to the stunningly irrational conclusion that it is somehow unsafe to *give* blood, with the result that blood banks are below normal in many cities. The news that the medical establishment considers AIDS a relatively difficult disease to catch has, rather than reassuring people, made them suspicious of their doctors, according to Dr. Thomas Plaut, assistant chief of behavioral sciences for the research branch at the National Institute of Mental Health. He might have had in mind Darlynn Spizzeri, a New York City mother who said she was keeping her child out of school because "we are afraid our children will catch the disease even if those so-called, quote-unquote experts say it is impossible."

The New York boycott probably looked more impressive on television than it deserved to be; it affected only two of the city's 32 community school boards, and the great majority of students went to school as usual. But the protesting parents are also suing the city, and a state Supreme Court justice began hearing arguments last week on what sort of danger a child with AIDS really poses to her classmates. The city based its decision on guidelines from the Centers for Disease Control, in Atlanta. The head of CDC's AIDS task force, Dr. James Curran, holds that there is no reason to exclude AIDS children from school unless "they are very ill themselves, can't control their behavior or their body fluids." Most children, of course, would rather bite their brothers and sisters than almost anyone else, yet CDC researchers have not found a single instance ("so far," they add cautiously) in which the disease was transmitted from one sibling to another. This is true even among children who were incubating the virus for years before anyone knew they were sick and therefore took no special precautions to avoid spreading it.

The boycotting parents found more persuasive the testimony of a local internist, Dr. Ronald Rosenblatt, who has treated a few

AIDS patients but has done no research in the field. As the first witness called in the hearing, Rosenblatt testified that there is "a definite possibility" the disease could be transmitted by blood from a cut or a nosebleed, by vomit or by "sharing a bologna sandwich." (Most leading authorities would agree that there is a possibility, but hardly a distinct one.) An acknowledged expert on children with AIDS, Dr. Arye Rubinstein, testified for the parents—under subpoena—the second day. He was not openly opposed to having the child in school, but he thought the city was wrong to keep her identity a secret from other parents and teachers. But school officials hold that identifying a child as having AIDS is for practical purposes the same as locking her out. The second grader in question was actually one of four New York AIDS patients of school age; one of the others is too sick to go to school and is being tutored in the hospital, and one is in a hospital because the child has nowhere else to live but will go to school when and if a foster home is found. And one child, whose identity became known last year, was taken out of school at the time out of fear of what officials described as "psychological damage" from harassment.

Dr. David Cohn, assistant director of Denver Disease Control, calls this "the leper syndrome." (Denver has two two-year-olds with a preliminary form of the disease known as "AIDS-related complex.") It was the leper syndrome that kept an eight-year-old hemophiliac who contracted AIDS through contaminated blood from starting third grade in Carmel, Calif., this fall. The school district is working with county health officials, the National Hemophilia Foundation and Stanford University hospital to educate teachers, parents and other students in hopes of creating what Superintendent Robert Infelise calls "a more accepting climate." Infelise says he "believes we're heading in that direction," although he isn't sure they will ever get there. In Swansea, Mass., a town of 15,000, 700 parents packed a three-hour meeting to hear doctors and school officials defend their decision to admit a 13-year-old AIDS patient. "It absolutely is the right thing to do," says Superintendent John E. McCarthy, adding, "People keep telling me I'm courageous."

It is likely that more parents and school boards will be facing these questions in the years ahead. There are only about 52 children with AIDS in the nation now—those surviving out of the total of 165 cases diagnosed—and the number of new cases resulting from transfusions should decline with the safeguards in place against contaminated blood. But most of the cases represent children who were born to a mother with AIDS, a category that seems likely to grow with the spread of the disease among intravenous drug users. The relative handful of problems seen so far may be dwarfed once these children reach school age—even allowing for the fact that some of them never will reach school age.

Schools of course are only one of the institutions affected. The fear of AIDS has spread to hospitals, although there are no documented cases of a health worker who caught AIDS from a patient, even among the hundreds who accidentally pricked themselves with used hypodermic needles or came in contact with body fluids. Four nurses at San Francisco General nevertheless filed a job-safety complaint because the hospital did not allow them to wear gloves or masks in dealing with most AIDS patients. An expert testifying for the hospital said that patients whose nurses wear protective clothing "feel like contaminated rats." The fear has spread to morticians, although the CDC says that the only precautions required in handling AIDS victims are those already in effect with victims of infectious blood diseases such as hepatitis virus B. Don Miller, a Baltimore gay activist who has AIDS, called 99 morticians and told them he had the disease and wanted to make advance funeral arrangements; 10 refused to handle him at all and half of the others set various conditions, such as requiring a sealed casket or refusing to embalm the body. The fear has spread to the Pentagon, which just two weeks ago announced that it would begin screening all new recruits next month for exposure to the AIDS virus—and rejecting those who test positive.

The fear seemed to grow stronger with the discovery that the virus may be excreted in tears. "Somehow," observes Anthony Fauci, director of the National Institute of Allergy and Infectious Diseases, "that sprang a fear that it must be all over the place"—although no one is known to have caught the disease from tears, and most experts agree that they are a highly inefficient form of transmission. The most important advance in AIDS research thus far—the development of a test for exposure to the virus—has done little to calm fears, but added a lot of fuel to the calls for society to take action to protect itself. Researchers have known all along that many more people have been exposed to the virus than have developed the disease. The usual figure is that 10 percent of those who have been infected will actually come down with AIDS, although some doctors believe that over time that proportion will grow. Those who have the virus without the disease are capable of spreading it, however; indeed, they may actually be the real threat because they are likely to have sex.

But until the blood test became available just last March, there was no way to identify who these carriers might be. Now there is, and though the test is not always reliable because it frequently yields a false positive result, the Pentagon, the Moral Majority and a growing number of life-insurance companies are interested in it. The Rev. Jerry Falwell, who two years ago described AIDS as divine retribution on homosexuals, has become alarmed at the discovery that it is no longer confined to those who he thinks deserve it. Among other steps, he has urged that AIDS blood tests be required during routine physical examinations and that positive results be reported to state boards of health. He also wants to make it a crime for individuals with AIDS to have sexual relations. It was in response to proposals such as this that Rep. Henry Waxman (California Democrat) plans to introduce a bill to prevent outsiders from discovering the results of the AIDS tests given to all blood donors.

The insurance industry wants to avoid the enormous potential liability for life and health coverage of AIDS patients, in the same way that it excludes, say, drug addicts and hemophiliacs. Stephen Rish, a vice president of Nationwide Insurance, says that "we would maintain . . . that anyone who would test positive for the virus would be uninsurable." Rather than test all applicants, though, the company will look for applicants in high-risk groups. A history of sexually transmitted disease would be one clue; so would naming an unrelated male as the policy beneficiary. An executive for another large insurance company suggested that male fashion designers and hairdressers will get extra scrutiny. The insurance question is fast becoming a major political issue; it is one of the most visible symbols right now of what homosexuals see as the growing threat to their civil rights posed by the AIDS panic. Three states—California, Florida and Wisconsin—have passed laws to prohibit insurance companies from requiring an AIDS blood test.

The point to remember is that as many as 2 million people may have been exposed to the virus—a number that continues to grow. As far as is known, anyone infected by the AIDS virus is infected for life and capable of passing it on through sexual contact; so potentially 1 adult American out of 100 represents the threat of lethal disease to anyone he (or she) takes to bed. The risk is much higher, of course, in the cities where AIDS cases are concentrated, such as New York, Los Angeles and Miami. It has been established that women can indeed catch AIDS through sexual relations with a man; the reverse happens also, although much less frequently. One result has been to spur the sale of condoms, which offer some protection; Concord Chemists, a busy pharmacy in midtown New York, reports that sales are up more than 30 percent in just three months—and that the majority of sales now are to women. Another result, which shows up in interviews if not yet in statistics, has been to make people cautious about having casual sex with strangers. Says Sally Dodds, president of the board of the Health Crisis Network in Miami: "People are asking themselves, is it worth dying to have sex with this person?"

The answer, of course, is sometimes yes. AIDS is a disease that cuts to the quick of people's most intense fears and desires, and that is why it exerts such a powerful force over us; even drug addicts sometimes resist the simple precaution of using sterile syringes because of the powerful emotional element involved in sharing a needle. Can 2 million people give up sex for the rest of their lives? Can they be forced to do so if they choose not to? Public-health officials have broad authority to quarantine people with dangerous illnesses, but their powers do not lend themselves well to the fight against AIDS. Occasionally a person with tuberculosis will refuse to take his medicine and have to be locked up, but usually only for a couple of weeks, after which he is no longer contagious. To completely control AIDS, notes Benjamin, the Alameda County health official, "you would have to quarantine people for life."

Will that ever be done? Not to all 2 million (or 500,000, or whatever the number is) carriers, surely. But what about the Alameda County AIDS patient who has sex with three to five men a week? "There are people like him everywhere," says Benjamin, explaining why the county health department decided it made little sense to quarantine one individual out of so many. Dr. Dean F. Echenberg, director of San Francisco's Bureau of Communicable Diseases, also argues against quarantine because, unlike, say, tuberculosis, which can be spread by coughing, "AIDS is spread through a consensual act." Does someone who has sexual relations with a stranger implicitly consent to the risk of contracting a lethal disease? Harvard's Curran doesn't think so; he is designing a model law to be used against someone who willfully spreads infection. It would call first for a form of voluntary control, such as signing an agreement to inform his partners that he has AIDS. "If he keeps returning with gonorrhea, if he admits that he can't change his behavior or if officials receive reports to that effect, then quarantine is in order," Curran says. He advocates a scale of progressively more stringent confinement, from daily check-in to an overnight hostel to full-time custody in a guarded hospital. Says Curran: "This is a plague and a menace, and I see nothing wrong with quarantine on a constitutional level."

He is right, of course: AIDS is a plague and a menace and a potential social disaster. But what about the second grader in New York—is she a menace? Psychologists who have studied the growing panic over AIDS agree that the problem is the public's desire for absolutes: parents don't want a course in epidemiology, they want someone to tell them that there is *no possible way* for AIDS to spread to their children. If they applied the same logic to the question of the school boiler blowing up, schools would be cold all winter. Medical science holds few certainties, and those are usually the bad news; we are going to have to learn to assess the risk of AIDS the way we do any other disease and weigh it against our obligations to our fellow citizens. If suspicion and fear get the better of us, it could tear our society apart—and the ravages of AIDS will be doubled by the damage we inflict on ourselves.

INSURERS TOO ARE AFRAID OF AIDS[5]

Along with its other consequences, AIDS could damage life insurance companies. The disease generally takes the lives of men in their 20s, 30s, and 40s, people the insurers depend on to be

[5]Reprint of a staffwritten article. Reprinted by permission from *Fortune*, p. 127. S. 15, '86. Copyright © 1985 by *Fortune*.

alive and paying premiums for many years to come. Moreover, revising the actuarial tables on which rates are based is a slow process. Current tables have not yet accounted for AIDS.

Insurers say they should be allowed to screen life insurance applicants from high-risk groups by testing for the AIDS virus. But such testing has provoked outcries from homosexuals and civil rights activists. In California, where insurers are not allowed to use results of tests for AIDS virus antibodies, some companies have resorted to a less precise—and less fair—method of judging whether an applicant is an AIDS risk. They use what are called lifestyle clues. Naming an unrelated male as the policy beneficiary is one clue. Several companies have told their representatives to be wary of applications from single males in large cities.

Great Republic Insurance Co. of Santa Barbara, California, tried to protect itself from AIDS-related claims by requiring a special questionnaire of all unmarried men in occupations that the company says have a high incidence of AIDS cases— restaurant employees, antique dealers, interior decorators, florists, and fashion industry workers. The questionnaire asks whether an applicant has had a recent weight loss, a sexually transmitted disease or immune disorder, or any "deviation from good health during the past six months." The National Gay Rights Advocates, based in San Francisco, sued Great Republic, claiming the company discriminated against homosexual men. Now Great Republic is moving to a new policy: asking all applicants identical questions regarding symptoms of, or treatment for, AIDS or ARC.

Screening has become a hot political issue. In the District of Columbia the insurance industry spent $200,000 on a media campaign opposing a bill to ban the use of AIDS testing by insurance companies. The D.C. council passed the bill anyway, and soon afterward a good many insurance companies stopped taking new business in the district. "The economic risk is huge," says Herbert L. De Prenger, president of Geico's life insurance affiliates. "We are not willing to bet our company just to stay in a small market."

Life insurers have a case for using the blood test to screen applicants. For one thing, the companies can be vulnerable to fraud since no state allows them to deny death benefits to a policyholder who lied on his application, provided the policy has been in effect for a minimum period, usually two years. "Also health insurers can always raise premiums, but life insurers cannot adjust their rates," says Peter Groom, an attorney in the California insurance department. "If people die off sooner than they're supposed to, it doesn't take long before the small life insurance company is severely imperiled."

AIDS worries health insurance companies too, of course, and they also try to screen out applicants who seem risky. Eleven states have created risk pools that guarantee coverage to people whose applications for health insurance were refused. The pools take in people with all sorts of problems, not just those who appear to be at risk for AIDS. Premiums under such pooling arrangements run to about 150% of the average rates for individuals.

That seems a reasonable solution to Willis Goldbeck, director of the Washington Business Group on Health, a nonprofit organization with quite a few Fortune 500 companies among its members. He feels, however, that screening to reduce risk raises questions about the nature of the insurance industry. Says he: "The principle of insurance is to spread risk. But insurance companies want to exclude from the risk pool those who are especially risky." Counters Stephen Rish, vice president of Nationwide Life Insurance Co. of Columbus, Ohio: "Insurance companies are businesses. They are not a social system."

FRIGHTEN AND BE FIRED[6]

The one good thing about AIDS is that its spread can be checked by specific acts of human, mainly sexual, self-discipline. The main bad thing about the Justice Department's ruling on the right of employers to discriminate against people with AIDS is that it slides away from this undisputed fact, into areas where prejudice may prevail.

The Justice Department had been asked by colleagues at the Department of Health and Human Services to decide whether the 1973 law that prohibits job discrimination against a handicapped person applies to people who either have AIDS (acquired immune deficiency syndrome) or have been exposed to the AIDS

[6]Reprinted by permission from *The Economist*, pp. 29–30, Je. 28, '86. Copyright © 1986 by *The Economist*.

virus. The assistant attorney-general's opinion, delivered on June 20th, was that the anti-discrimination law applies to the disabling effects of AIDS but not to the fear of contagion. What this means in practice is that an employer may not sack somebody on the ground that he is disabled by AIDS but may sack him on the ground that he is thought to be infectious to his fellow-employees.

The spectre of a plague-like contagion is implicit in this opinion, which was substituted for a less tendentious draft prepared by the Justice Department's career staff but rejected by their political masters. Dr. Robert Windom, the new assistant secretary for health, responded swiftly by stressing that no evidence suggests that the AIDS virus is spread through the sort of casual contact that occurs at work, in schools or in similar settings. Dr. James Mason, the director of the Centres for Disease Control, added that there is no evidence of the disease being transmitted within a family (except to sexual partners or to children born to infected mothers) and strong evidence that there is no danger of catching AIDS through sneezing or coughing.

In the five years of the disease's documentation, 22,000 people in America have caught AIDS and more than half of them, 12,000, are already dead. A tenfold increase, and more, is expected in the next five years; the projection is that by 1991 America will have had 270,000 cases and nearly 180,000 deaths. Most of these future victims already have the virus in their blood. It is estimated that 1m–1.5m Americans are infected and that about a quarter of them will come down with the disease within the next five years.

Against these bleak figures, and in the absence, as yet, of any effective treatment or vaccine, the only tool for checking the spread of the disease is public education. The virus is transmitted through blood or semen or a mixture of the two. Nearly three-quarters of the sufferers are homosexual or bisexual men and about a quarter are intravenous drug users (with overlapping between the two groups); about 7% are heterosexual men and women, a proportion that is rising quite fast. The goal, propagated by teachers, doctors and many of the people at risk, is to avoid sexual promiscuity and, in particular, unchecked anal intercourse; to observe elementary rules of hygiene, including the use of a clean needle for drug takers; and, probably, to undergo the blood test that shows whether or not somebody has been exposed to the virus.

Suspects are less likely to allow their blood to be tested if, in the present climate of opinion, they run the chance of losing their jobs if the results turn out to be positive: people with the virus in their blood are often as infectious as those with the most deadly of symptoms. If the Justice Department's opinion were to be accepted, somebody who reacted positively to the test, but without having the AIDS symptoms, would be even more vulnerable to dismissal than somebody, disabled by AIDS, who could at least argue for the protection of the law.

The department's ruling applies only to jobs paid for partly or wholly by the federal government. But, although individual states write their own rules on the treatment of handicapped people, they traditionally accept a lead from the federal government on matters to do with civil rights and discrimination.

The department's opinion could be challenged if and when a clutch of pending cases reach the courts. In Florida, for instance, an argument has been going on about whether the dismissal of a county budget analyst, who suffers from AIDS, breaks the state's handicap law. And the Supreme Court will be receiving briefs early next month in an analogous case, also from Florida; it concerns a teacher with tuberculosis, dismissed not because of her illness, which would be against the law, but because of her ability to transmit the disease, which, her employers claim, is not covered by the law. A different case could come from California. An initiative promoted by followers of Mr. Lyndon LaRouche has now gathered enough signatures to go on the ballot in November; it would control the movements of victims and carriers of AIDS. [EDITOR'S NOTE: The Lyndon LaRouche–sponsored Proposition 64 was defeated in the November '86 election by 73% of the voters.]

The damage done by the Justice Department's ruling is not that it raises the question of contagion but that, by its way of doing so, it nourishes the unsubstantiated belief that AIDS can be caught from casual contact in office, store or cafeteria. This confuses the issue. The disease is fearful enough without the extra cruelty of a policy which, if followed through to the end, could make more than a million not-yet-sick people unemployable.

AIDS IN THE WORKPLACE[7]

One of this century's most serious epidemics seems about to spread into the political realm. Last week, even as more than 2,000 researchers from at least 41 nations were gathering in Paris to pool all current scientific knowledge about AIDS, the medical issues were overshadowed by news from the United States. In Washington the Justice Department ruled that some employers may legally fire AIDS victims if their motive is to protect other workers—despite doctors' assurances that the disease cannot be spread through casual contact. And in California a proposal to give state officials broad powers to contain the disease—including quarantine—was certified for submission to the voters in November. The initiative, sponsored by followers of political extremist Lyndon LaRouche, will provide the first electoral response to AIDS since it began its frightening global spread five years ago. [EDITOR'S NOTE: Proposition 64 was defeated in the California election, with 73% of the electorate voting against it.]

The new federal ruling resolves a heated dispute within the government: whether AIDS victims are handicapped persons as defined by the Rehabilitation Act of 1973. This law prohibits discrimination against the handicapped in federal agencies and in organizations such as universities and hospitals that receive federal funds. In a 49-page opinion, which the executive branch is bound to follow in dealing with complaints of discrimination, Assistant Attorney General Charles J. Cooper wrote that discrimination based on the physical disability caused by AIDS might be a violation of the law. But, he added, "the statute does not restrict measures taken to prevent the spread of the disease." The result is an anomaly of sorts: an AIDS victim whose abilities are impaired may have protection against dismissal, but a fully functioning AIDS carrier may not—as long as dismissal is based on a fear of contagion. The ruling suggested an AIDS carrier wouldn't qualify as "handicapped," and hence would have no legal basis for challenging discriminatory acts under the 1973 statute.

Medical evidence: The ruling was promptly attacked by gay-rights activists. "Implicit in the . . . policy is [the idea] that there

[7]Reprint of an article by Matt Clark, *Newsweek* staffwriter. Reprinted by permission from *Newsweek*, 106:82-3. Jl. 7, '86. Copyright © 1986 by *Newsweek*.

is some kind of health basis to believe that AIDS is likely to be transmitted in the workplace," said American Civil Liberties Union attorney Nan Hunter. "That is outlandish based on the medical evidence." In addition, Hunter and others fear that the ruling could lead to mandatory testing of all workers in federally funded employment. Whether such testing, currently being done among military recruits, would be a violation of constitutional rights has never been settled in court. But at least some of the questions raised by the opinion itself could be resolved by the Supreme Court as early as next year. The justices have agreed to hear a case raising the question of whether the 1973 law protects victims of tuberculosis. The ACLU hopes to get the court to include the AIDS issue in its deliberations.

In California the question of AIDS discrimination will be decided by voters rather than judges. In another of its recent surprises, the LaRouche organization collected 683,000 signatures—nearly double the number required—to place a measure on the ballot that would put AIDS in the same category of infectious disease as measles or TB—and authorize health officers to use the full range of their protective powers.

The proposal was roundly denounced by the California Medical Association, the Los Angeles City Council and Los Angeles Mayor Tom Bradley, who is the Democratic candidate for governor. Bradley asked his Republican opponent to join him in calling the measure "a throwback to the Dark Ages." The initiative is the first real test of the emotional impact of AIDS on the average voter. Political experts expect the measure to suffer the same fate that a state initiative barring gay schoolteachers did in 1978—defeat, but only after a costly public-relations battle.

Even if it weren't a political and legal issue, the AIDS picture is grim enough. About 30,000 cases have been officially counted around the world, two-thirds of them in the United States. But at the second International Conference on AIDS in Paris last week, Halfand Mahler of the World Health Organization noted that AIDS is a largely hidden disease and estimated that 100,000 was a more realistic figure. It has been reported in 92 countries, he noted (and a delegate from the Soviet Union said that a few cases had occurred in his country). "In recent history," he said, "there is hardly any disease that has taken humanity in its grip as AIDS has."

Out of Africa: The picture of AIDS in Africa, where the disease apparently started and where it strikes men and women in equal proportion, is worse than epidemiologists have thought. Dr. Bela Kapita of Mama Yemo Hospital in Kinshasa, Zaire, who has treated 1,000 victims, more than any physician in the world, said that 6 percent of all people in the sub-Sahara zone are infected, and the number is increasing by 1 percent each year. While the disease was once thought to be concentrated in central and eastern Africa, he noted, it appears to be spreading rapidly throughout the continent—"from Algeria to South Africa."

What experts fear the most is that the African situation may be a harbinger of things to come elsewhere. "This virus doesn't know if a person's homosexual or heterosexual," noted Dr. James Curran of the U.S. Centers for Disease Control. And, indeed, one of the more disturbing reports at the conference pointed to an increase in the spread of AIDS among heterosexuals. Reporting on blood-test results among 304,000 U.S. Army volunteers, Col. Donald Burke of the Walter Reed Army Institute of Research noted that 1.56 per 1,000 men showed signs of infection, as did women at a rate of .62 per 1,000. This amounts to a 2.5–1 male-to-female ratio of AIDS infection among volunteers, which contrasts sharply against the 13–1 ratio for previously reported cases in this country. And in most of New York City, Burke said, the male–female ratio of AIDS infection among recruits is close to one to one. No one can be sure, of course, how many of the Army volunteers fall into the well-known risk groups, mostly male homosexuals and intravenous drug users. But these findings support the idea—shared by many epidemiologists—that AIDS can be transmitted between the sexes and could become an even more serious health threat than it already is.

IV. THE FUTURE

EDITOR'S INTRODUCTION

Although the AIDS outlook is uncertain, the scientific community is not sanguine about the immediate future. Projections that have proved accurate in the past point to an alarming escalation of the disease, with 235,000 new cases expected by 1991. By then 179,000 deaths from AIDS are also foreseen. These estimates are based partly on the likelihood that between one and two million people in the U. S. have already been exposed to the virus and carry it in their systems. Of these, perhaps twenty percent or more will contract the disease. But this figure may be conservative. On the average, AIDS takes two to five years before it develops, but it could take much longer, and the incidence of AIDS in five years might dwarf the projections. Troubling, too, is the uncertainty over the possible incidence of AIDS in heterosexuals. In Africa AIDS is apparently spread chiefly among heterosexuals, and there is an undercurrent of anxiety that the AIDS virus might mutate, becoming more common in the heterosexual population than it has been thus far.

In the first article in this section, Deborah M. Barnes, writing in *Science* magazine, reviews the grim projections for the AIDS epidemic through 1991. And in a lengthy symposium article appearing in *Harper's*, a group of experts exchange their views on AIDS. Part of their debate concerns the federal government's inadequate response to this national health crisis, the politics of AIDS, changing lifestyles, and a host of civil rights issues. Although this symposium was published before the Surgeon General's Report, the panelists concur with its findings, that a massive campaign must be undertaken to educate the public about the risks of sexual promiscuity. With a threat as great as AIDS, no one should act in ignorance.

GRIM PROJECTIONS FOR AIDS EPIDEMIC[1]

During the first 5 years of the AIDS epidemic, approximately 35,000 people in the United States will have developed the disease. Over the next 5 years, the Public Health Service (PHS) estimates that about 235,000 new cases will occur. Scientists attending a recent planning session on AIDS (acquired immune deficiency syndrome) that led to the PHS report generally agree with these estimates. But what is really uncertain is how many people will become infected with the AIDS virus over the next 5 years and who those people will be, issues the report does not address.

Most of the people who will develop the full disease in the next 5 years are infected with the virus now, a number many participants of the recent meeting at the Coolfont resort in West Virginia believe is 1 to 1.5 million. How many of those infected will go on to develop the disease in uncertain, but the PHS report indicates that the conversion rate from being infected with the AIDS virus to having the full disease is between 20% and 30%. However, scientists at Coolfont noted that this rate is difficult to predict and that it varies according to different studies.

These uncertainties also leave open the question of projected medical costs for AIDS, perhaps underestimated by acting assistant secretary for health Donald MacDonald, who puts it at $8 billion to $16 billion in the year 1991. MacDonald spoke about the PHS report at a recent press conference in Washington, DC.

Another major question concerns who in the United States is likely to become infected with the AIDS virus during the next 5 years. Mounting evidence indicates that it is no longer appropriate to speak in terms of high-risk groups for AIDS. Rather, "the risk for becoming infected with the AIDS virus is really a behavior," according to Anthony Fauci of the National Institute of Allergy and Infectious Diseases. "The risk for AIDS is having sex with someone who is infected or being exposed to blood that is infected. The risk is not being a homosexual man or being a member of any group."

[1]Reprint of an article by Deborah M. Barnes, *Science* staffwriter. Reprinted by permission from *Science*, 1589–90. Je. 27, '86. Copyright © 1986 by *Science*.

Nevertheless, the great majority of Americans infected today are either homosexual men or intravenous drug users, populations that overlap to different degrees in different parts of the country. Because about three-quarters of the people who will develop full AIDS by 1991 are already infected with the virus, most AIDS patients in 5 years will be either homosexual men or intravenous drug users. Still, the projected number of cases of AIDS among heterosexuals is increasing at a slightly higher rate than among those now considered to be at risk for the disease.

More than 80 physicians and scientists from government and academic laboratories, government health policy–makers and analysts, epidemiologists, a government attorney, and physicians in private practice participated in the recent Coolfont conference. There were no representatives of private industry. Conference participants emphasized that, in order to meet AIDS-related health care demands over the next 5 years, government, academia, and industry must expand existing collaborative research efforts, but no specific proposals were made. Their deliberations and conclusions provided the basis for the new PHS document.

All of the numerical projections contained in the PHS report were prepared by the Centers for Disease Control (CDC) from a mathematical model based on extrapolations of previous data. Speaking at the Coolfont meeting, James Curran and Meade Morgan of the CDC indicated that their estimates were much more likely to be accurate over the next 2 years than over longer periods of time.

They predict that by the end of this year 35,000 persons will have been diagnosed as having AIDS, with 16,000 new cases in 1986 alone. By 1991, according to the new projections, the cumulative total will reach 201,000 to 311,000, with 74,000 new cases diagnosed in that year alone. Some 18,000 people will have died from AIDS by December of 1986 (9000 of whom will die this year). The number of deaths is projected to rise to 54,000 in 1991, for a cumulative total of 179,000 deaths at the end of the next 5-year period. The number of children with AIDS will probably increase tenfold over the next 5 years, from over 300 today to more than 3000 in 1991.

There is no way to determine accurately how many people will become infected with the AIDS virus over the next 5 years. "Even the current data are soft," notes Morgan. Because of these uncertainties, "I'm personally very uncomfortable with projections of the incidence of infection," says Curran. The recent PHS projections therefore contain no estimate of the number of infected individuals by the year 1991.

Nevertheless, the number of infected people and those sick with AIDS will increase dramatically over the next 5 years, leading MacDonald to characterize the projected medical costs as "staggering." Health care costs for AIDS patients are based upon the number of people with the disease who receive direct medical care and the average medical cost per patient. MacDonald estimates that "in 1991 the medical care of AIDS patients will require between $8 billion and $16 billion," figures that do not include home care given by friends or family or lost income due to illness.

This PHS projection is based on the assumption that the average cost per patient will be about $46,000, a figure derived largely from health care costs for AIDS patients in the San Francisco area. Some participants at the Coolfont meeting called this estimate unrealistically low because the gay community in San Francisco provides support and home care assistance for AIDS patients, making their average cost much lower than the national average. However, Walter Dowdle, acting AIDS coordinator for PHS, thinks the $46,000 figure is realistic because "it has been shown to be achievable and we hope that by 1991 there will be better treatments for AIDS."

The AIDS virus is transmitted in three major ways—by sexual contact, through contaminated blood or blood products, and to children born to infected mothers. The virus is present in blood, semen, vaginal secretions, saliva, sweat, tears, and various body tissues including brain and skin. It is most commonly associated with cells, such as infected T lymphocytes or macrophages, and the role of cell-free transmission of virus is unclear at present.

The predominant method of transmission of the AIDS virus is through sexual contact with someone who is infected, either a man or a woman. At the Coolfont meeting, Thomas Zuck of the Food and Drug Administration (FDA) said, "We need to tell people what behaviors put them at high risk for the disease." It is not only having multiple sexual partners that puts an individual at risk, it is also having sex with someone who has multiple sexual partners that is risky.

People who become infected with the AIDS virus make antibodies to different parts of the virus, its outer envelope and inner core, for example. Screening a person for viral infection means testing for seropositivity, or having these antibodies in the blood. Researchers think that individuals are probably most contagious early in the course of their infection before they develop the full disease. Thus, most people probably become infected with the AIDS virus by having sex with seemingly healthy partners.

Scientists are working to develop vaccines to prevent infection by the AIDS virus and antiviral drugs to treat persons already infected. The new PHS report indicates that a vaccine will probably not be available for general use in this decade, but that "limited clinical testing for some [vaccines] could begin within 2 years." The report also indicates that "a safe and effective antiviral agent is not likely to be in use for the next several years."

The PHS report reflects the opinions of Coolfont participants in its approach to health care policy. Both stress the importance of massive educational programs targeted at special populations, including children and teenagers, women, and minority groups, as well as the general population. In addition, AIDS screening and counseling centers should be established throughout the country. Use of these centers would be voluntary and information would be confidential. Anyone found to be infected with the virus would be strongly encouraged to notify his or her sexual contacts and refer them to a center for screening.

At present, state and local health services are largely unequipped to cope with sharply rising numbers of persons infected with the AIDS virus or sick with the full disease. The magnitude of the problem calls for a coordinated response from federal, state, and local agencies; greatly expanded educational and training programs for health care workers; and careful assessment of the appropriate care and costs for care required at various stages of the disease.

AIDS: WHAT IS TO BE DONE?[2]

When a mysterious contagion known as Acquired Immunodeficiency Syndrome began to kill large numbers of people a few years ago, various

[2]Reprint of a symposium article, *Harper's*. Reprinted by permission from *Harper's*, 271:39–52. O. '85. Copyright © 1985 by *Harper's*.

moral authorities took solace in the observation that its victims, most of whom were homosexuals or drug addicts, seemed well chosen for divine retribution. Confronted with a lethal and seemingly unappeasable plague, enlightened man found himself grateful to discover a reassuring semblance of the wrath of God.

As the numbers continued to mount and it became undeniable that even the morally immaculate were among the afflicted—as they had been from the beginning—it grew increasingly difficult to consign AIDS to its accustomed place as a pestilence of the lower depths. Only when Rock Hudson's illness became known did the disease achieve the status of a full-fledged "social problem." But the confirmation that viruses remain unimpressed by human pieties did not address the issue of how to slow the spread of a deadly and still puzzling disease.

What exactly do we know about AIDS? Given that knowledge, how can the state marshall a response while protecting the rights of the disenfranchised groups that have been most affected? *Harper's* recently invited a group of public health officials, physicians, scientists, and medical historians to consider what can be done to contain a modern plague.

The following Forum is based on a discussion held at the Princeton Club in New York City. Jonathan Lieberson served as moderator.

JONATHAN LIEBERSON is contributing editor of *New York Review of Books* and an associate at the Population Council, an organization concerned with social scientific and biomedical research on population and development.

MERVYN F. SILVERMAN is a consultant to local governments and private organizations on AIDS and other health issues. From 1977 to January 1985 he was director of health for the city and county of San Francisco.

MATHILDE KRIM is chairperson of the board of trustees of the AIDS Medical Foundation and former head of the interferon laboratory at the Sloan-Kettering Institute for Cancer Research.

RONALD BAYER is an associate for policy studies at the Hastings Center and co-director of the center's Project on AIDS, Public Health, and Civil Liberties.

GERALD FRIEDLAND is director of Medical Service 1 at Montefiore Medical Center in New York City and an associate professor of medicine at Albert Einstein College of Medicine. He supervises the care of many AIDS patients and conducts clinical and epidemiological research into how the disease is transmitted.

GARY MACDONALD is executive director of the AIDS Action Council of the Federation of AIDS-Related Organizations, a Washington, D.C., lobbying group that represents local organizations providing a wide range of support services.

ANN GIUDICI FETTNER writes about AIDS for the *New York Native*. She was senior health adviser to the government of Kenya from 1977 to 1980. A revised edition of her book *The Truth about AIDS* will be published in October.

STEPHEN SCHULTZ is deputy commissioner for epidemiologic services at the New York City Health Department and oversees the department's research on AIDS.

ALLAN M. BRANDT is an assistant professor of the history of medicine and science at Harvard Medical School and the author of *No Magic Bullet: A Social History of Venereal Disease in the United States since 1880.*

MATHEW J. SHEBAR was director of legal services for Gay Men's Health Crisis. He is the author of *The Gay Men's Health Crisis Attorneys' Manual.* His forthcoming book, *Lowenstein's Protégé*, describes his experiences representing people with AIDS.

JONATHAN LIEBERSON: As everyone is aware by now, AIDS continues to run its appalling course. At the beginning of 1981, the year AIDS was first recognized, there were fewer than sixty cases in the United States; since then, there have been more than 12,000. Every day more and more people are diagnosed as having a lethal condition for which, as yet, there seems to be no effective treatment.

In view of the gravity of this situation, our task today is to review the facts about the epidemic and to discuss what factors influence society's response to it. What precisely is known, and not known, about AIDS? Have its cause and the means by which it is transmitted been definitely established? Is there reason to expect that it will increasingly affect people in groups that have remained largely unaffected? Are researchers close to finding a cure or an effective treatment for AIDS?

Second, what policies should the United States and other nations adopt in dealing with this epidemic? What in fact *has* been done by the U.S. government thus far? What principles should guide public discussion of ways to control and contain the epidemic? Under what conditions should we consider using measures that may raise troubling issues of privacy, confidentiality, and civil rights? Has the government's response been greatly influenced, as many charge, by the fact that most of those afflicted with AIDS are homosexuals or drug addicts?

Finally, how has society responded to AIDS? How will it respond as the number of patients continues to rise? And how will the spread of AIDS influence sexual attitudes in general?

Dr. Silverman, how many people are currently afflicted with AIDS, who are they, and how fast is it spreading?

MERVYN F. SILVERMAN: As of August 12, 12,408 people in the United States had been reported as having AIDS; 6,212 had died. The number of cases is roughly doubling every year, but it is doubling within certain well-defined "high-risk" groups which emerged early on in the epidemic. According to the Centers for Disease Control in Atlanta, gay and bisexual men constitute 73 percent of AIDS patients nationwide; intravenous drug abusers make up 17 percent; transfusion recipients 2 percent; and hemophiliacs one percent. Heterosexuals who have had sexual contact with members of high-risk groups make up another one percent, and the remaining AIDS cases are classified as "noncharacteristic." It is expected there will be more than 30,000 cases by the end of 1986.

MATHILDE KRIM: It should be emphasized that these figures include only cases of the disease as defined by the CDC. This narrow definition applies to a relatively small proportion of cases within a much larger population of diseased people. Those numbers, however frightening, represent the tip of the iceberg.

The condition now known as AIDS was first recognized in 1981 when an unusual form of pneumonia, *Pneumocystis carinii*, killed five young men in Los Angeles. All five were homosexual and suffered from a profound impairment of their immune systems. In particular, they lacked T-4 lymphocytes, a type of white blood cell that is essential to defending the body against infections. As the number of cases began to grow, physicians saw this pattern repeated: all people with AIDS had a severely impaired immune system that left them vulnerable to rare "opportunistic" infections and cancers, particularly Kaposi's sarcoma. This association of different diseases, several of which often strike the same patient simultaneously, constitutes a "syndrome." The conglomeration of illnesses was apparently made possible by an underlying immunodeficiency that the heretofore healthy patients had somehow "acquired." Thus, Acquired Immunodeficiency Syndrome, or AIDS.

For two years, researchers focused on identifying the cause of the immune deficiency. Meanwhile, the CDC's nationwide surveillance showed that the disease was concentrated in the high-risk groups Dr. Silverman named. Researchers noted that members of these groups tend to be exposed to various infections or allogeneic cells—such as foreign blood cells or sperm—both of which can damage the immune system; some even speculated that AIDS might simply be an extreme result of this damage. But other researchers believed an infectious agent might be involved.

In April 1984, Dr. Luc Montagnier's group at the Pasteur Institute in Paris isolated a virus that he called "lymphadenopathy-associated virus," or LAV, because it had been found in a patient with chronically swollen lymph glands. Less than a year later, Dr. Robert Gallo of the National Institutes of Health isolated a virus from an AIDS patient that he called "human T-cell lymphotrophic virus, type three," or HTLV-III. The two viruses were later found to be virtually identical, and thus the virus now thought to cause—or at least be one cause of—AIDS is known as LAV/HTLV-III.

LIEBERSON: But AIDS patients are susceptible to all sorts of infections. What proof is there that this particular virus *causes* the disease?

KRIM: LAV/HTLV-III has a strong predilection for infecting and growing in T-4 cells when studied in the laboratory. And it has been found in virtually all patients suffering from AIDS itself or from the lesser forms of the disease that don't fit the CDC definition.

Dr. Gallo's group was able to develop a blood test, called the ELISA test, which indicates whether someone has been exposed to the virus. This test does not detect disease, only the antibodies formed when someone has been exposed to LAV/HTLV-III. But it can be used to screen contaminated blood from the blood supply and to estimate the spread of the virus. For example, surveys show that in New York City, as many as 80 percent of IV drug users, as many as 60 percent of healthy gay men, and one out of every thousand healthy blood donors have been infected. These numbers probably vary from city to city, but the CDC has estimated that a million people might already have been infected nationwide.

While infection with the virus seems necessary for the occurrence of AIDS, it isn't clear whether it's sufficient to cause it. The great majority of those with the virus as yet show no symptoms. On the other hand, the incubation period for AIDS may be very long, from several months to more than five years. Meanwhile, many who *are* sick are not considered to have AIDS. According to the CDC's definition, one must not only show an acquired immune deficiency but be afflicted with one or more of certain specified opportunistic infections, or with certain cancers. Yet many infected people exhibit a broad range of symptoms, from persistent low-grade fever, unexplained weight loss, and swollen lymph glands to various degrees of immune deficiency sometimes associated with infections and cancers other than those specified by the CDC.

LIEBERSON: Would it be correct to refer to these manifestations as "pre-AIDS," as some have?

KRIM: No, "pre-AIDS" implies that these symptoms inevitably lead to AIDS. Yet many patients have had them for several years and have not gone on to develop AIDS. The symptoms constitute a condition that is now referred to as AIDS-related complex, or ARC. There may be ten ARC patients for every one AIDS patient.

RONALD BAYER: Current estimates are that between 5 percent and 20 percent of those infected with LAV/HTLV-III will go on to develop AIDS-related complex or AIDS within the next five years. This means there might eventually be as many as 200,000 terribly ill people in this country.

KRIM: The problem with those percentages is that we have not followed any of these infected people for more than about five years. Since AIDS can take so long to appear after infection, the percentage of those infected who will develop the full-blown syndrome may be much higher than we think. And of course as we speak, the million Americans who are infected are going about the business of transmitting the virus—studies show that at least two thirds of those with the virus are capable of infecting others. So there may well be many more than 200,000 cases.

GERALD FRIEDLAND: What often happens with a new disease is that the lethal cases—the most dramatic ones—are counted first. Yet these represent only the top of a pyramid beneath which extend a majority of infected people who exhibit a broad spectrum of symptoms, or none at all. Because AIDS is such a new disease, the ratio of asymptomatic infection to mild disease to serious disease to lethal disease isn't clear. The 5 percent to 20 percent estimate is based on the current epidemiological evidence. Yet, as Dr. Krim said, the incubation period could be much longer than the disease's history itself. The virus could get into a cell and remain dormant. And then, ten or fifteen years later, some biostress might cause it to manifest itself. But we can't know yet, because we are *making* history now.

SILVERMAN: What makes the virus manifest itself? Each of the stages between the mildest sign of LAV/HTLV-III infection—which may simply be a positive blood test—and AIDS as defined by the CDC represents a greater deterioration of the immune system. In order to develop any of these manifestations, or perhaps even to be infected in the first place, a co-factor of some sort is probably necessary. Since those who develop the disease fall into groups that tend to have compromised immune systems, an existing weakness in the immune system seems the most likely co-factor.

By shooting up for years, IV drug abusers have destroyed, or at least attacked, their immune systems. People who need blood transfusions tend to be in very difficult straits and probably have weakened immune systems, as do hemophiliacs, who receive blood products from thousands of people during their lifetime.

LIEBERSON: But why have homosexuals constituted the majority of cases from the beginning? And what is meant by "homosexual" here? What kind of homosexual? What groups?

GARY MACDONALD: Good Lord, are there more than ten kinds? We should have invited Dr. Kinsey. "Gay or bisexual men" refers to a group of males, largely between the ages of twenty and fifty, who have sex with other males.

LIEBERSON: I wasn't looking for a definition of homosexuality. Given the fact that members of the high-risk groups tend to have pre-existing immune deficiencies, are we speaking about any homosexual, or only those who engage in certain practices?

SILVERMAN: Gay men tend to have compromised immune systems for a couple of reasons. First, semen is known to be immunosuppressive when it is introduced into the bloodstream through breaks in mucous membranes. Second, gay men, especially "fast-lane" gays who have many sexual partners, generally have a lot of infections, which weaken their immune systems.

KRIM: Certain sexual acts also seem to facilitate transmission of the virus. In particular, anal-receptive intercourse may facilitate both transmission—by letting infected sperm into the bloodstream—and an immunological reaction to that sperm.

MACDONALD: Look, I think the moment may have arrived to desexualize this disease. AIDS is *not* a "gay disease," despite its epidemiology. Yet we homosexualize it, and by so doing end up posing the wrong questions. There is no evidence to support the notion that gay men in general are immunocompromised *because* they engage in anal intercourse, despite the fact that semen itself may be immunosuppressive in some circumstances. And gay men have been doing this for centuries with no dire results.

Isn't the point really that an infectious agent has been introduced into the gay male population and, because gay men tend to have sex with each other, is spreading there? There is nothing inherent in being gay that promotes the disease; after all, the number of cases within each high-risk group appears to be increasing at the same rate. AIDS is not transmitted because of who you *are*, but because of what you *do*. From the beginning, 17 percent of AIDS patients have been IV drug users, and at least 6 percent have never fit into any of the high-risk groups. In New Jersey, the *majority* of AIDS patients are IV drug users. By concentrating on gay and bisexual men, people are able to ignore the fact that this disease has been present in what has charmingly come to be called "the general population" *from the beginning*. It was not spread from one of the other groups. It was *there*.

FRIEDLAND: The majority of our patients in the Bronx are IV drug users, and a quarter are women who have contracted the disease either by using dirty needles or by having sex with infected men.

ANN GIUDICI FETTNER: And the CDC admits that at least 10 percent of AIDS sufferers are gay *and* use IV drugs. Yet they are automatically counted in the homosexual and bisexual men category, regardless of what might be known—or not known—about how they became infected.

In their desire to keep AIDS in its place as a "gay disease," people ignore the fact that in Central Africa the sexual spread of the disease occurs almost solely among heterosexuals; slightly more women than men are infected. At the university hospital in Kinshasa, the capital of Zaire, three or four AIDS cases are coming in every day. Interestingly enough, in some places where the virus is prevalent, there is virtually no disease. For example, scientists have found that as many as 51 percent of the people in some remote tribes in northern Kenya are infected—but there's no AIDS. They're finding the virus in green monkeys in Zaire as well, yet they don't seem to be sick.

SILVERMAN: It's possible that the virus has existed in animals for a long time and has only recently mutated and begun to infect humans. Or it may have been present in humans in isolated regions of Africa for years. Perhaps it began to spread as more roads were built and people moved to the cities. Today, jet travel can spread a disease around the world almost instantly.

MACDONALD: The outbreak in Western Europe seems to be following the American model: the largest group affected is gay and bisexual men, followed by IV drug users, and then heterosexuals. The number of cases is increasing rapidly, particularly in France and West Germany.

LIEBERSON: What precisely do we know about how the disease is spread?

KRIM: The virus is probably not spread by casual contact—kissing or living in the same household or sitting near someone on a bus. But it *is* transmissible sexually and through the blood. It is less contagious than hepatitis or flu.

SILVERMAN: People seem to think AIDS is some virus from a Steven Spielberg movie—a supervirus. Well, it isn't. Soap and water destroy it. In fact, LAV/HTLV-III is sexually transmitted precisely because it is so fragile.

LIEBERSON: Does "sexually transmitted" mean that a person who has sex with someone who has the virus is likely to get it?

FRIEDLAND: Frankly, we have no idea how likely it is that the virus would be transmitted during any single sexual encounter. Someone may have to be exposed several times to be infected.

STEPHEN SCHULTZ: We know the virus is present in body fluids, but we don't know which of them are effective transmitters. Just because the virus is found in saliva doesn't mean saliva transmits it. Many public health officials have taken the conservative approach and assumed that if the virus is present in *any* body fluid, every attempt should be made to avoid spreading it around.

FRIEDLAND: To obtain *biological* proof of how the virus is transmitted, as opposed to epidemiological proof—which is essentially circumstantial evidence—we would have to take infected body fluids, inject them into subjects, and wait for infection to occur. Since this is impossible to do in humans, researchers must find an animal that can become infected with the virus and duplicate the disease. Work in this area began only recently. Today, we can only make admittedly circumstantial assumptions about how the virus is transmitted.

SILVERMAN: Epidemiologically speaking, one could say that semen appears more likely to transmit the virus than saliva. The two factors associated with transmission seem to be multiple sex partners, which suggests that a number of exposures might be necessary, and anal-receptive intercourse, which suggests that semen is a likely transmitter.

FRIEDLAND: The cleaner epidemiologic information derived from transfusion studies confirms that blood can transmit the virus. In some cases, the original blood donors of people who have acquired the disease have been located, and the virus in their blood isolated. These transfusion studies give us our most reliable evidence about the disease's incubation period. The multiple sexual encounters of many gay and bisexual men, for example, or the numerous episodes of needle-sharing among drug addicts, usually make it impossible to determine when infection occurred.

BAYER: Although we can retrospectively trace cases back to blood donors, we don't know how many recipients of that blood did *not* become infected. Not everyone given a transfusion with infected blood develops antibodies.

SILVERMAN: Retrospective studies of any disease usually give us fairly definite information about transmission. But with AIDS, we're just now building that body of information.

MACDONALD: Still, there are *no* data suggesting the virus is transmissible by casual contact or through saliva. If it were, we would undoubtedly be seeing a markedly greater number of cases than we have so far.

SILVERMAN: And the numbers of AIDS patients, though doubling every year, are doubling *within* the high-risk groups. No mothers of AIDS patients have gotten it, for example.

KRIM: An even stronger argument is that there has been no recorded transmission of the virus between AIDS patients and medical personnel.

SILVERMAN: The point is that AIDS is predominantly a sexually transmitted disease, and that means it's a *behavioral* disease. People who *don't* do certain things very likely will not get it. People who *do* do certain things risk getting it.

KRIM: This means that the infection—and therefore AIDS—is essentially preventable, not by medical means as yet but by changing how people behave. People must be taught how to protect themselves from getting the virus. That is the great failing of our government: it has made no real effort to provide this education.

ALLAN M. BRANDT: That raises the question of how very rational fears of what is after all a terrifying disease can be separated from the powerful, irrational fears that are spreading across the country. Despite the scientific uncertainty, emerging epidemiological data tell us a good deal about why we need not fear AIDS under certain circumstances. Yet this information has gotten lost in the public portrayal of the disease.

SCHULTZ: Look at the press, which has been pointing its finger at prostitutes and warning heterosexuals that they run a "grave risk" of catching AIDS. The cover of *Life* proclaimed "Now No One Is Safe from AIDS" in big red letters. Meanwhile, the government warns that *everyone* must be careful, which, while literally true, tends to worry people unduly. The evidence that AIDS is spreading outside the high-risk groups, beyond the percentage of "noncharacteristic" cases we've *always* seen, is negligible.

MACDONALD: Only because the gay aspect of the disease has been so sensationalized can people say, four years after the epidemic broke out, my goodness, *heterosexuals* are at risk too. The disease *seems* to have "broken out" in the general population, but that's only because we have not really talked about AIDS before—its epidemiology, modes of transmission, and so on. Before, when discussing AIDS, we were really talking about attitudes toward homosexuality, or something else altogether.

SILVERMAN: Only one percent of all AIDS cases can definitely be traced to sexual transmission between men and women. But this might be changing. Eighty-six percent of AIDS patients in San Francisco are homosexual or bisexual men who are not IV drug abusers—as opposed to 59 percent in New York City. But the percentage of IV drug abusers in San Francisco who are infected seems to be rising. If a man has sex with a woman who has contracted the virus by using dirty needles, he could become infected. So we may start seeing more cases among heterosexuals in San Francisco.

FETTNER: The press keeps talking about hookers—how they get it from dirty needles and spread it to their customers. But do we know exactly *how* they spread it?

FRIEDLAND: We *know* the virus is transmissible through blood, and almost any body fluid can be contaminated by blood. A woman's gums may be bleeding when she kisses her partner; maybe cells are exchanged that are infected with the virus. Or her vaginal fluids may contain it. At this point, we just don't know.

I treat many women who have contracted AIDS through sex with men, and as far as we can determine, these women seldom engage in anal-receptive sex. Many have longstanding relationships—with a single infected person. A simple formula might be: the more frequent the sexual activity, gay or straight, with an infected partner, and the more body fluids exchanged, the more likely it is that the virus will be transmitted.

SILVERMAN: The clearest rule is: prevent the exchange of body fluids. Those with multiple partners—and especially members of high-risk groups—should use condoms, and use them properly. People in these groups can have safe sex so long as they are honest with each other and take the proper precautions. And there are certainly erotic and exciting sexual activities that do not entail an exchange of body fluids. Use your imagination.

FETTNER: Use your imagination? What kind of educational message is that?

SILVERMAN: Well, statistical studies, particularly those being conducted in San Francisco, show that this advice is being followed. We hear constantly about the "promiscuity" of gays and the shocking bathhouses, but few people mention the phenomenal change in behavior that has taken place within the gay community since the AIDS crisis began. The rate of rectal gonorrhea has plummeted, falling more than 75 percent.

LIEBERSON: What are the prospects for developing a cure or an effective treatment for this disease?

KRIM: There are three rather disquieting obstacles to developing an effective vaccine or treatment. First, LAV/HTLV-III is a retrovirus, a very particular kind of virus unknown in humans until a few years ago. Such a virus has genetic material composed of double-stranded RNA that must be transcribed into DNA by a viral enzyme. The viral DNA is then integrated into human chromosomes. Once it is there, nothing can remove it—infection is lifelong, and the virus reproduces at a very rapid rate. At best, treatment might succeed in suppressing multiplication of the virus.

Second, although this virus induces the production of antibodies, these antibodies almost never succeed in neutralizing it. The immunological reaction against infection is not generally effective.

Finally, this virus, like flu viruses, seems to mutate—to modify its genetic structure—frequently. This raises the question of whether an effective vaccine—or at least a single effective vaccine—can ever be developed. It's quite possible that an antibody that works against one strain of the virus might be powerless against another strain, which is exactly the difficulty we have in developing a flu vaccine.

So LAV/HTLV-III infects a person for life; it remains infectious despite the presence of antibodies produced to combat it; and developing a vaccine will be very difficult, and may be impossible. And we have learned through bitter experience that treating patients in the terminal stage of this infection is futile.

FRIEDLAND: I wince when I hear that. I spend most of my time treating patients; to say we have no cure is not to say we do nothing. We are unable to cure many diseases; so we concentrate on palliating them. We do many things to improve the quality of life of AIDS patients. Every day we learn more about how to recognize the opportunistic infections early and to treat them effectively.

KRIM: But AIDS is a lethal disease, and at this point most patients die of it within a couple of years. There is now a clear consensus among researchers that treatment aimed at suppressing the multiplication of the virus and at stimulating and restoring the immune system should be undertaken earlier, not only prior to the development of the cancers and opportunistic infections but prior to the development of any significant immune deficiency—if possible, immediately after infection with LAV/HTLV-III.

But there is a problem—the current pharmacopoeia is devoid of drugs that can do these things. Some rare drugs such as HPA-23, Suramin, and Ribavirin seem to inhibit retrovirus multiplication in animals or in the laboratory, but investigators have only begun to study how effective they might be against LAV/HTLV-III in man—and how toxic they are. Meanwhile, drugs able to restore immune functions simply don't exist.

One would expect that very assertive and organized research into these areas would be under way. Unfortunately, our government in its wisdom has done little or nothing to fund such research. Work on antiviral drugs was started only this year, and the government has made available very, very little money to pay for it. Research on the use of interferons, which are known to be effective against retroviruses in animals, has been left entirely to the pharmaceutical companies that produce them.

MACDONALD: It's obvious that the government was caught off guard and is still off guard. The federal government in general—and the Public Health Service in particular—is not equipped to respond to such a devastating epidemic. That has not really changed since the polio epidemic in the 1950s. Not enough money is allocated, and the various agencies of the Public Health Service compete for the money that is, frequently duplicating work or not performing it at all because they misunderstand which agency is supposed to do what. I hope the AIDS epidemic will point up the extent to which we need to examine the role of our government in public health emergencies.

When a disease is controversial or politically sensitive, politicians and federal officials are even more hesitant to take an assertive role. From the beginning, AIDS was a political issue more than a medical one, and it remains so today. When officials discuss AIDS, they are usually not discussing a disease but the people who suffer from it, and how voters react to it.

FETTNER: Federal agencies have been forceful in leading efforts in prevention, screening, and treatment of other diseases, yet they have done very little with respect to AIDS. The government has done literally nothing in the way of education, and yet, as Dr. Krim said, our only defense against this disease is to educate people about how they can avoid infection. The Department of Health and Human Services has allocated only $120,000 this year for public education—*down* from $200,000 last year.

MACDONALD: The truth is that the federal government does not want to be in the position of talking about gay sex acts—which is what it would have to do to mount an effective educational campaign.

MATHEW J. SHEBAR: In fact, twenty-four states still have laws prohibiting sodomy, specifically the act of anal penetration. So the federal government might be condoning criminal activity in those states if it began telling men to use condoms when having sex with other men.

SILVERMAN: The government only has to provide funds so that communities can educate their people about AIDS in whatever way they deem most effective.

MACDONALD: But that presupposes the government believes it *has* a role in these matters—which it apparently does not. The standard procedure of the Public Health Service when it is confronted with an epidemic is to determine the cause and develop a vaccine. The federal government has not taken responsibility for funding AIDS treatment or education because these elements don't appear in that model. Up to now, it has responded to AIDS by working to discover its cause and by pushing forward a crash program to develop a vaccine. Even the greatly increased funds that the government proposes to spend on education next year will be administered by officials who do not believe in the efficacy of prevention.

Yet consider the cost of this epidemic. According to the CDC, the average cost per diagnosed case is about $140,000. For the first 9,000 cases, the cost in health care alone has been about $1.25 billion, some 60 percent of which has been public money. And it is sure to cost much more this year.

SILVERMAN: The cost per case in San Francisco is probably half that figure. San Francisco is spending about $4 million this year on outpatient services for AIDS patients. The idea is to reduce the hospital stay and care for patients in their homes with skilled nurses and other support staff. The average hospital stay in San Francisco for an AIDS patient is about eleven days, which is much less than in New York.

This system reduces total AIDS expenditures immensely. But it's enormously costly for the local government, because charges are not reimbursed by Medicaid or other programs. Yet the federal government considers the provision of these services a local responsibility, even though they reduce total costs. Meanwhile, New York and San Francisco, because of the quality of care they provide, now attract AIDS patients from across the country.

BAYER: The fact is that our health care system doesn't provide adequate care for large numbers of people. How can we provide money for long-term care for AIDS patients? We can't provide it for the elderly or the homeless.

SHEBAR: The whole question of federal involvement is a double-edged sword, particularly when it comes to prevention programs. Asked how to "prevent" AIDS, the man on the street might demand rather draconian measures. Some right-wing spokesmen have already advocated the mandatory quarantine of AIDS patients. Officials in the Reagan Administration might believe they're being rather evenhanded when it comes to AIDS: Well, they say, we may not be giving much money to those gays for education, but at least we're not locking them up, as Jerry Falwell keeps demanding.

SCHULTZ: Those on the radical right aren't the only ones talking about quarantine; so are many people in the public health profession.

FETTNER: Quarantine is not some sort of paranoid gay fantasy. James Mason, head of the CDC and acting assistant secretary for health, has conceded that it has been discussed by federal officials.

KRIM: A quarantine would not only be terribly cruel and harmful, but also completely counterproductive. After all, the only people who could be forcibly committed to a hospital are diagnosed AIDS patients showing clinical symptoms. Yet these people are very ill, and they are usually not interested in sex. And the more advanced their condition, the less infectious they become.

The people most likely to infect others with the virus are those who have been infected but do not evidence symptoms. They think of themselves as healthy; for all we know, they may never get sick.

SILVERMAN: Besides the obvious ethical issues this raises, if we tried to lock up all those infected, we would have to imprison upward of a million people, most of whom are not sick. And how would we identify the infected people? My God, we would have to give everyone in the country a blood test, and isolate all those who tested positive—some of whom, of course, would test *false*-positive.

BAYER: It's clear mass quarantine couldn't work, at least not in a way that would benefit public health; but it would have a profound effect on civil liberties. Many less extreme measures have also been discussed, and because they are more plausible, they are even more troubling.

For example, some have proposed mandatory screening for AIDS in schools, in the military, in places of employment. It's not unreasonable to expect that many who are deeply concerned about public health—and not necessarily right-wingers—will begin to discuss this possibility. If nothing else, such a discussion might help us confront the fact that in some sense we have lost the ability to consider "the public" when we debate public health issues. The concern for privacy, civil liberties, and constitutional rights has become so pre-eminent in the past few decades that it is impossible to determine at what point these individual protections might be compromised in the name of public health.

SILVERMAN: I disagree. Officials must simply look at these issues logically and intelligently. If they do, they'll see, for example, that there is no real point in mandatory mass screening. The disease is not casually spread, so there is no reason for an employer to screen his employees, except perhaps to avoid paying out insurance money.

The military already screens all blood it collects on its bases. Commanding officers are informed when someone tests positive for LAV/HTLV-III—apparently not for health reasons, but so he may be discharged for being a homosexual.

SHEBAR: If the military discharges someone because he has AIDS, it has violated the law. But if it discharges someone—on the basis of the same test—because he is a homosexual, it's within the law.

MACDONALD: But the test is often inaccurate, and in any case, a positive test doesn't indicate a person has the disease. It only shows that the immune system has been exposed to the virus and has built up antibodies to fight it.

In New Jersey it was recently proposed that anyone giving blood whose antibody test was positive be informed, and that blood banks be required to report test results to the state. But certainly the government should intervene only when it can do something constructive. What can it do for someone who tests positive?

BAYER: It is not unreasonable to assume that once public health officials notified someone that he had tested positive, he would have a moral obligation to behave prudently when he had sexual contact with others.

MACDONALD: But a test result is not required to give that message to members of high-risk groups.

SILVERMAN: Well, it definitely makes that message more effective. That's why I'm in favor of people in high-risk groups—gays and bisexuals, IV drug abusers—taking the blood test. Someone who has a positive test can at least come in for counseling. What do we tell him? First, the evidence indicates that a large percentage of people carrying the virus will *not* get AIDS. Second, there are steps you can take to help ensure that you stay healthy. Above all, build up your immune system: follow a good diet, get a lot of rest and exercise. Most important, make sure you don't expose yourself to the virus again—and, for God's sake, don't expose anyone else.

To someone who tests negative, we can offer advice on how to stay that way: build up the immune system and behave in ways that don't increase the risk of exposure. And, as Dr. Krim mentioned, if we begin treating people at an earlier stage of the infection, we may be able to accomplish something with treatment.

LIEBERSON: What's the possibility of the test indicating someone has the virus when he doesn't?

FRIEDLAND: Any test has its "false-positive" rate. In screening IV drug users in New York City—up to 80 percent of whom may have the virus—the test should be pretty reliable. But if you're screening a population that has a relatively *low* frequency of infection, the test's false-positive rate may actually be higher than the true rate of infection of the group. So a given positive test is more likely to be false-positive than it is to indicate infection. This is why it's problematic to screen large numbers of people who are unlikely to be infected.

BAYER: But more elaborate confirmatory tests like the Western Blot have been developed, and they are very reliable. When such tests are used, the rate of false-positives is negligible.

SCHULTZ: However accurate the test, many argue that if effective treatment for the disease isn't available, then screening people is immoral. Between the wars, the United States screened much of its population for syphilis—but it had only a very ineffective therapy to offer.

BRANDT: Premarital screening for syphilis has been mandatory in most states for years, and we know now that test results in the past were often false-positives. Yet many people who tested positive were not allowed to marry until they received highly toxic treatment.

It's interesting that Dr. Silverman said we should tell people who test positive to behave in a certain way, and people who test negative to behave in a certain way—the same way, in fact. That suggests to me that the main purpose of testing people would be to frighten them, rather than to offer them effective treatment. Government officials, physicians, and others have traditionally hoped that fear of venereal disease would prevent it—by preventing "illicit" sex. But historically, fear has never been enough to prevent venereal disease.

SILVERMAN: Well, fear has been one hell of an effective motivator in the gay community. Yet our statistics show that the change in behavior has been quantitative rather than qualitative: people have reduced the number of their sexual partners, but some have not changed their sexual activity, at least not to the same extent. But sex with three people today may provide as much exposure as sex with a dozen people did three years ago, because so many more gay men are now infected—one out of two in San Francisco.

I concede that screening—and I mean voluntary screening, not mandatory—can be misused. But I believe it can be effective as an educational tool—just like showing a smoker an X-ray of his lungs.

SHEBAR: Behind such cynicism must lie the hope that *everyone* in the gay community will test positive—what a great motivator that would be! Among our clients at the Gay Men's Health Crisis Center who committed suicide, three times as many were suffering from ARC as from AIDS itself. It's the waiting, the checking for symptoms every day, that's so terrible. Every cold seems like a sign of the end.

The blood test does not diagnose disease. It does not suggest any treatment. And it is extraordinarily dangerous in its implications for civil rights. Last summer, I got a call from a man who had been given an annual physical by his employer—a Fortune 500 pharmaceutical corporation—and had been tested without his knowledge for the LAV/HTLV-III antibody. His employer—not a physician—called him in, told him he had tested positive for the antibody, and summarily fired him. This man had no idea what the test meant. I helped him get his job back and have the test result deleted from his medical records.

SILVERMAN: To prevent such abuses, California just passed a law forbidding use of the test in screening employees or insurance applicants.

MACDONALD: The implications of mass screening are frightening. When a bureaucracy like the Public Health Service is given a very simple task—and screening blood is a very simple task—it tends to reduce a complex phenomenon to very simple formulas: if someone tests positive, thus and thus is true; if someone tests negative, thus and thus is true. The bureaucracy doesn't pay attention to whether anything is really being accomplished. Look at the Red Cross's policy of sending people with confirmed positive results to their physicians. Their physicians can't *do* anything.

FETTNER: The Red Cross is also putting the names of those who test positive on a list.

BAYER: Blood banks always maintain something called a deferral directory, which lists anyone whose blood has been rejected for medical or other reasons. Its purpose is basically to screen out blood that may not be safe.

Of course any kind of list, whatever its purpose, presents a problem. The Red Cross list presents a particular problem for those who believe that individuals should *not* be notified of positive results because they might be terrified by information that is not necessarily accurate.

At present, a blood donor is notified only if both the ELISA screen test and the confirmatory Western Blot test are positive. If someone tests positively on the ELISA but negatively on the Western Blot, his blood is not used and his name appears on the deferral list—but he is not notified. This list presents the problem, especially since no computer list can be absolutely confidential. Are health care professionals ethically bound to tell people their names are on the list, even though it has not been confirmed that they have the antibody?

Almost everyone acknowledges that many gay men want to take the test, whether it will mean their names end up on a list or not. That's why people are worried that members of high-risk groups will flock to donate blood in order to get the test results, and thereby risk infecting the blood supply. So now we are in the strange position of spending public money to set up testing centers while acknowledging that the test can't give much useful information.

SHEBAR: Creating alternative centers has to be done. But gay leaders should be sending out a clear message that people should *not* take the test, both to ensure that high-risk people don't flock to blood banks and to protect their rights.

SILVERMAN: In California, people can take the test anonymously, which is one way to mitigate the confidentiality problem.

SCHULTZ: Anonymous testing intended to let people find out their antibody status, so that those who have the virus can choose to have sex only with others who have it, might be effective as a preventive measure. But the program being tried on the West Coast, and apparently favored by the federal government, uses testing as a means to trace the sexual contacts of those who are infected, and to frighten them into severely curtailing their sexual activity. As Mr. Brandt said, this is the traditional approach to VD. But without an effective treatment to offer, the chances of getting people to cooperate with such a program are dubious.

Government's ability to alter sexual behavior has always been very limited.

LIEBERSON: We heard earlier that some observers expect 30,000 cases of AIDS by the end of 1986. What kind of social response can we expect in the next few years?

MACDONALD: There will be a wave of hysteria as people become aware of the scope of the epidemic.

BAYER: "Hysteria" gives the impression that people's fears are utterly groundless, but 30,000 cases of a lethal, infectious disease seem a rather good reason to be worried. At the least, AIDS will generate a crisis in our health care systems. The isolation rooms at municipal hospitals like Bellevue are already devoted almost exclusively to AIDS cases.

SHEBAR: If the progress of this disease is not impeded, it will devastate our cities. The future of AIDS is already here; it exists in our prisons. In these closed areas, where hygiene is poor, unconsenting homosexuality rampant, and IV drug abuse widespread, the disease is spreading unchecked. In New York State prisons, about 200 AIDS cases have already been reported, and the state has announced plans to spend $7.5 million on a new AIDS prison treatment center; as it is, patients are literally chained to their beds in prison hospitals. Our prisons can be thought of as a sort of dirty mirror of our urban centers.

BRANDT: But how will the government and the press address people's fears? If they are addressed in an irrational way, they could lead to policies most people would regret. The main problem is ignorance. We understand, for example, that a positive blood test doesn't mean someone has AIDS. But the press has distorted that fact enormously. And such distortions create an atmosphere in which scapegoating thrives.

BAYER: Although some AIDS patients have lost their jobs or lost their insurance, a well-organized group of lawyers and other advocates from the gay community and civil liberties groups has thus far managed to keep in check what might have been a profoundly irrational public response. The CDC has even negotiated with gay leaders about the conditions under which AIDS research would be done.

But as the cases mount, will such cooperation begin to break down? How many "liberal" values—the right to privacy and confidentiality, the civil rights won during the past decade or two by vulnerable minorities—might be eroded or even swept away by hysteria over AIDS?

MACDONALD: The high-risk groups—primarily gay and bisexual men—have borne the brunt of not only the disease itself but the political costs of marshaling a measured public response to it. Believe me, we would like nothing better than to withdraw from the role of principal advocate for the victims of this disease and become participants in a general response. The gay community has been unfairly cast as the adversary from the beginning. AIDS was dubbed "the gay plague," which evokes the image of irresponsible, promiscuous deviants living on the fringes of society and infecting the body politic with a dread disease. That conception of AIDS prevails in most of this country to this day.

BAYER: But the disease does constitute a plague for the gay community, especially if as many as 20 percent of those with the virus will go on to develop the disease.

BRANDT: The point is that AIDS is an important *social* problem. The press screams that *now* babies are getting it—as if the gays had it first. In doing so, the "innocent" victims are divided from the "guilty." Such an attitude has been a traditional part of our reaction to venereal disease. In the early twentieth century one spoke of *venereul insontium*—children who got it congenitally, wives who caught it from unfaithful husbands. There has always been a desire to separate "innocent" from "guilty." But all are victims.

LIEBERSON: Perhaps one way of looking at that distinction follows from Dr. Silverman's point that AIDS is a behavioral disease—certain people put themselves at risk and do so knowingly, while others don't. A baby doesn't. Neither does an unconscious person who has been in an auto accident and needs a transfusion.

SILVERMAN: If somebody behaves in an unsafe way *today*, he is not innocent. But the fact that gay men had sex without taking precautions five years ago doesn't make them guilty of anything. This disease could conceivably have been spread primarily through heterosexual activities—would that have made the general population "guilty"? Everyone was innocent—until we knew how to protect ourselves.

MACDONALD: We should realize, however self-serving this sounds, that were it not for the gay community fighting this tooth and nail with the government and everyone else, we wouldn't know what we do now—there would not *be* a response to AIDS.

FETTNER: That's indisputable. Even today there is no highly placed official in the federal government who realizes the need to educate people about the disease.

SHEBAR: Margaret Heckler, secretary of health and human services, said last April that she fears it's spreading to "the community at large." I call her the secretary of health and heterosexual services.

SILVERMAN: But there is a Catch-22 in the gay community's response. Gays have been the only ones loudly advocating a strong public effort to fight the disease—but in so doing they have attracted all the attention and all the animosity.

SHEBAR: Yet as the AIDS panic grows and gay leaders present themselves more and more responsibly, more people may realize that gays are a minority whose rights deserve to be legally protected. And the millions of closeted homosexuals in this country might be encouraged to come out and declare themselves gay.

FRIEDLAND: I want to point out that among AIDS patients, gays alone have the power to organize. Although IV drug users represent almost a fifth of those with AIDS nationwide, they obviously can't demand help from the government as an organized group.

BRANDT: In Canada, where sanitary needles are widely available, the number of IV drug users with AIDS is very low. But in the United States, addicts share needles—and transmit disease—

because it is so difficult to obtain them. By making it easier to obtain sanitary needles, the government could take a decisive step toward reducing the spread of the virus among IV drug users—and their sexual contacts.

Yet despite all the hysteria, many people still dismiss the crisis by saying: "It's only gays and drug addicts. Who needs them anyway?"

FRIEDLAND: Those people *should* be concerned, if for no other reason than that IV drug users are the most likely people to transmit AIDS outside their own at-risk group.

FETTNER: Another problem in rallying public concern is the large number of blacks with the disease. Nationwide, a quarter of all AIDS patients are black.

BAYER: That the groups affected are largely disenfranchised raises that question again: How does one fashion a vigorous public health response while at the same time acknowledging the importance of protecting privacy and civil liberties? Frankly, I don't believe privacy and civil liberties are compatible with such a vigorous response. If we continue to claim that they are, we may find ourselves with policies that ignore civil liberties altogether.

MACDONALD: We must remember that when public health officials propose measures like screening, they are in effect proposing to a population already outside the law that something else be taken away. Homosexuals are an unprotected class, and you are suggesting doing something to this class in order to protect "the public's" health.

If Congress passed laws assuring the civil rights of gay people, or even mandating that all test results be confidential, that would be a different situation. But that is *not* the situation today.

BAYER: The cruel irony is that in the absence of those political guarantees, the gay community is put in the position of hesitating to agree to the very research necessary to respond to the disease effectively.

MACDONALD: I'm not aware of many instances where the gay community has resisted research. But it should be pointed out that most public health officials are oblivious to the true situation of gay people. A while back, a high-level Public Health Service official said to me: "Frankly, the best response to this disease would be for all gay men to settle down in monogamous relationships." This man seemed to believe that two gay men in Omaha could simply get married, retire to the suburbs, and drive their 2.4 cars happily for the rest of their lives.

SHEBAR: Today, gays in San Francisco are protected from the disease spreading through the bathhouses. Those bathhouses have been restricted, and most gays cooperated when the restrictions were imposed. Why? Because San Francisco has a gay rights bill and openly gay elected officials; gays there know that the director of health who imposed the restrictions, Mervyn Silverman, is not an enemy of gay people.

In New York City, there is no gay rights bill, there are no openly gay elected officials. Because of this, any regulation of the bathhouses has been resisted—I believe unwisely.

BAYER: Yet even in San Francisco, the gay community was split about closing the bathhouses.

SILVERMAN: That is a very complex issue. The bathhouses have served as social centers and, for some, as refuges; they are seen as symbols of gay liberation. Even though only 5 percent of San Francisco's gay population regularly frequented these establishments, there was great fear among gays that closing them would lead to increased oppression nationwide.

Our major goal was to motivate people to change their behavior, regardless of location. We couldn't risk letting a political controversy over the bathhouses overshadow the central message. We realized that message must be getting across when the VD rate began to drop dramatically. We then felt we could move against the baths. San Francisco was spending over $6 million to reduce the spread of this disease while bathhouse owners were making a profit by facilitating high-risk activities. After the baths were closed, more than half of my mail from the gay community supported the action.

LIEBERSON: What influence will the disease have on sexual mores and practices?

SILVERMAN: As the number of cases keeps growing, there will be a revolution—some would say a counterrevolution—in sexual attitudes and behavior. It won't bring us back to the Victorian era, but people will get to know each other a lot better before they jump into bed. After all, a considerable change in behavior accompanied the herpes scare, and herpes doesn't kill.

FETTNER: I see that change happening in my own family. My nineteen-year-old son is very gun-shy about sex. All of a sudden it may be deadly.

SHEBAR: I have a great hope that this epidemic might accomplish something magical—free gay men from the burden of anonymity. Gay men can maintain that anonymity only when they have their sex in underground places with people they don't know—or when they stay closeted, afraid to reveal who they really are. But because of AIDS, anonymous sex in the gay community has already decreased.

It must be recognized that there is a direct correlation between anonymity and oppression. When a parent discourages his gay son from becoming involved with another man; when a church refuses to accept gay congregants; when an employer says, "Just keep it out of the office"—what they are all really saying is, keep it *in* the bathhouses and backrooms, the places where one runs a higher risk of being infected. I think AIDS will lead gay people to rebel against this sort of oppression and to become more visibly committed to their gay identities and to their partners. Quite frankly, I believe gay marriage will be legal by the turn of the century. That couple in Omaha may be able to settle down in the suburbs someday.

BRANDT: I've heard too often that some disease is just what society needs to discourage promiscuity and bring about meaningful, caring relationships. The sexual counterrevolution didn't come with herpes, and it won't with AIDS—no matter how much some people hope it will.

FRIEDLAND: There is no evidence that AIDS has brought about any substantial change in the habits of drug users or caused a decrease in their numbers. In New York City there are 200,000 IV drug users, and anywhere from 40 percent to 87 percent of them—depending on which study you look at—are infected with the virus. Every day more young people are introduced to drugs, and exposed to the virus. There has been almost no response to this problem, either by community groups or public agencies.

KRIM: I don't understand why organizations concerned with family health are not worried about AIDS. Clearly we have reached a stage where there should be programs in every high school and college to explain to young people the dangers of drug abuse and casual sex. What exactly are we waiting for?

BIBLIOGRAPHY

An asterisk (*) preceding a reference indicates that the article or part of it has been reprinted in this book.

BOOKS AND PAMPHLETS

Altman, Dennis. AIDS in the mind of America. Doubleday. '86.

Baker, Janet. AIDS: everything you must know about acquired immune deficiency syndrome. R & E Publishers. '83.

Black, David. The plague years: a chronicle of AIDS, the epidemic of our times. Simon & Schuster. '86.

Cahill, Kevin, ed. The AIDS epidemic. St. Martin's Press. '83.

Cantwell, Alan, Jr. AIDS: the mystery and the solution. Aries Rising. '84.

DeVita, Vincent et al. AIDS: etiology, diagnosis, treatment, and prevention. Lippincott. '85.

Fettner, Ann Giudici and Check, William A. The truth about AIDS: evolution of an epidemic. Holt, Rinehart & Winston. '84.

Fisher, Richard B. AIDS: your questions answered. Alyson Publications. '84.

Friedman-Kien, Alvin E. and Lauberstein, Linda J., eds. AIDS: the epidemic of Kaposi's sarcoma and opportunistic infections. Masson. '84.

Gong, Victor, ed. Understanding AIDS: a comprehensive guide. Rutgers University Press. '85.

Gottlieb, Michael S. and Groopman, Jerome E. Acquired immune deficiency syndrome. A. R. Liss. '84.

Klein, Eva, ed. Acquired immune deficiency syndrome. S. Karger. '85.

Lieberson-Smith, Richard. The question of AIDS. Academy of Science. '85.

Nichols, Eve K. Mobilizing against AIDS: the unfinished story of a virus. Harvard University Press. '86.

Nichols, Stuart and Ostrow, David G. Psychiatric implications of acquired immune deficiency syndrome. American Psychiatric Association. '84.

Selikoff, Irving J. et al., eds. Acquired immune deficiency syndrome. New York Academy of Science. '84.

Smith, W. Henry. Plain words about AIDS. Whitefall Press. '85.

*U. S. Department of Health and Human Services. Surgeon general's report on acquired immune deficiency syndrome. '86.

Vaeth, J. M., ed. Cancer and AIDS. S. Karger. '85.

PERIODICALS

*My personal experience with AIDS. Ferrara, Anthony J. American Psychologist. pp. 1285-86. N. '84.

A crisis in public health. Leishman, Katie. Atlantic. 256:18-41. O. '85.

Fear and loathing in the workplace. Pave, Irene. Business Week. p. 126. N. 25, '85.

*'Fast-buck' artists are making a killing on AIDS. Ticer, Scott. Business Week. pp. 85-6. D. 2, '85.

AIDS on stage. Weales, Gerald. Commonweal. 112:406-7. Jl. 12, '85.

AIDS and the blood supply. Eckert, R. D. Consumer Research Magazine. 68:20-5. O. '85.

AIDS: epidemic of the '80s. Kupersmith, Judith. Dance Magazine. 60:76-80. Ja. '86.

AIDS: the quest for a cure. Langone, John. Discover. pp. 75-77. Ja. '85.

*AIDS: special report. Langone, John. Discover. 6:28-53. D. '85.

*'Look, doctor, I'm dying. Give me the drug.' Grady, Denise. Discover. pp. 78-86. Ag. '86.

AIDS update: still no reason for hysteria. Langone, John. Discover. pp. 28-47. S. '86.

Fear of dying. Economist. pp. 29-30. S. 14, '85.

A plague on all their houses? Economist. pp. 27-8. N. 2, '85.

Is nobody safe from AIDS? Economist. pp. 79-81. F. 1, '86.

*Frighten and be fired. Economist. pp. 29-30. Je. 28, '86.

The reasons behind blood donor screening. Miller, R. W. FDA Consumer. 19:31-4. N. '85.

*AIDS progress report. Hecht, Annabel. FDA Consumer. 20:32-5. F. '86.

AIDS to the rescue. Beauchamp, Marc. Forbes. pp. 72-4. N. 18, '85.

Bucking the bureaucrats. Forbes. 137:10-12. Mr. 24, '86.

Helping battle AIDS. Fiernan, Jaclyn. Fortune. pp. 57-8. Ap. 15, '85.

AIDS and business: problems of costs and compassion. Chapman, Fern Shumer. Fortune. pp. 122-7. S. 15, '86.

*Insurers too are afraid of AIDS. Fortune. p. 127. S. 15, '86.

Farewell, sexual revolution. Hello, new Victorianism. Cornish, E. S. Futurist. 20:24. Ja./F. '86.

AIDS: what women must know now! Zimmerman, D. R. and Gadsby, D. Good Housekeeping. 201:245-6. N. '85.

*AIDS: what is to be done? (symposium). Harper's. 271:39-52. O. '85.

AIDS hotline: is sex dead? Deutsch, G. Harper's Bazaar. 119:118+. Mr. '86.

The new victims. Barnes, E. and Hollister, A. Life. 8:12-19. Jl. '85.

French admit that cyclosporine as AIDS treatment failed to work. Los Angeles Times. Sec. I, p. 3. My. 7, '86.

AIDS epidemic sweeps through Uganda; experts say 10% of sexually active populace may be infected. Powers, Charles T. Los Angeles Times. Sec. I, p. 1. My. 24, '86.

Use of AZT by 6,000 AIDS victims okd. Los Angeles Times. Sec. I, p. 20. O. 1, '86.

Testing donors for AIDS. Finlayson, Ann. Maclean's. 98:49. My. 27, '85.

*The new terror of AIDS. Allen, Glen. Maclean's. 98:35. Ag. 12, '85.

*The pursuit of a cure. Ohlendorf, Pat. Maclean's. 98:36-7. Ag. 12, '85.

An epidemic of fear. Barber, John. Maclean's. 98:62-3. S. 23, '85.

Another AIDS treatment. Rogers, June. Maclean's. 98:61. N. 11, '85.

The ethics of AIDS. Allen, Glen. Maclean's. 98:44-8. N. 18, '85.

AIDS has both sexes running scared. Cantarow, E. Mademoiselle. 90:158-9+. F. '84.

AIDS is not for men only. Norwood, C. Mademoiselle. 91:198-9+. S. '85.

Inside the billion-dollar business of blood. Rock, A. Money. 15:152-4+. Mr. '86.

AIDS: neglect. Kaye, R. Nation. 236:627. My. 21, '83.

*A social disease. Editorial. Nation. 241:195-6. S. 14, '85.

Stigmatizing the victim. Editorial. Nation. 241:195-6. S. 14, '85.

Unleashing bias. Editorial. Nation. 242:34. Jl. 5/12, '86.

Journal of a plague year. Mano, D. K. National Review. 35:836-7. Jl. 8, '83.

The AIDS question. Buckley, W. F. National Review. 37:63. O. 18, '85.

AIDS, nature, and the nature of AIDS. National Review. 37:18. N. 1, '85.

AIDS update. Mano, D. K. National Review. 38:59-60. F. 14, '86.

The politicization of AIDS. Mano, D. K. National Review. 38:23. Mr. 28, '86.

The history of an epidemic. Bazell, Robert. New Republic. 189:14–18. Ag. 1, '83.

The politics of a plague. Krauthammer, Charles. New Republic. 189:18–21. Ag. 1, '83.

Waking up to AIDS. Bazell, Robert. New Republic. 192:17–19. My. 13, '85.

*Afraids. Editorial. New Republic. 193:7–8. O. 14, '85.

The politics of AIDS. Barnes, Fred. New Republic. 193:11–24. N. 4, '85.

*AIDS and lawyers. Huber, Peter. New Republic. 194:14–15. My. 5, '86.

How a virus that is very hard to catch crossed the world. Meldrum, Julian. New Statesman. pp. 14–5. S. '85.

The cry of 'The Normal Heart.' Smith, Dimitia. New York. 18:42–6. Je. 3, '85.

Insurance against AIDS. Blaun, Randi. New York. 62–5. Je. 3, '85.

The last word on avoiding AIDS. Tanne, Janice Hopkins. New York. 18:28–34. O. 7, '85.

Anatomy of an epidemic. Lieberson, Jonathan. New York Review of Books. 30:17–22. Ag. 18, '83.

The reality of AIDS. Lieberson, Jonathan. New York Review of Books. 32:43–8. Ja. 16, '86.

*Acquired immune deficiency syndrome: 100 questions and answers. New York State Department of Health booklet. N. 1, '86.

AIDS among prisoners poses a national problem. New York Times. Sec. I, p. 12. Ag. 11, '85.

Fright grips Brazil as AIDS cases suddenly rise. Riding, Alan. New York Times. Sec. I, p. 4. Ag. 25, '85.

Haitians go back on list of groups at risk for AIDS. New York Times. Sec. I, p. 2. Jl. 28, '86.

Cases of AIDS rise around the world; . . . disease now affects 74 countries. New York Times. Sec. I, p. 7. O. 5, '86.

Heterosexuals and AIDS: the concern is growing. Eckholm, Erik. New York Times. p. Cl, 7. O. 28, '86.

Federal efforts on AIDS criticized as gravely weak. New York Times. p. Al, 18. O. 30, '86.

Teaming up against AIDS. Hurt, M. New York Times Magazine. pp. 42–4+. Mr. 2, '86.

Tracing the origins of AIDS. Seligman, Jean. Newsweek. 103:101–2. My. 7, '84.

AIDS strikes a star. Gelman, D. Newsweek. 106:68–9. Ag. 5, '85.

*The AIDS conflict. Adler, Jerry. Newsweek. 106:18–24. S. 23, '85.

*Sins of omission. Alter, Jonathan. Newsweek. 106:25. S. 23, '85.

AIDS and civil rights. Press, A. Newsweek. 106:86+. N. 18, '85.

*AIDS in the workplace. Clark, Matt. Newsweek. 106:82-3. Jl. 7, '86.

Moving target: searching for a vaccine and a cure. Begley, S. Newsweek. 108:36. N. 24, '86.

Monkey AIDS. Gauntt, T. Omni. 6:22. Ap. '84.

Guidelines for enrolling children with AIDS set up in two states. Phi Delta Kappan. 66:448-9. F. '85.

New federal guidelines say children with AIDS can attend school. Phi Delta Kappan. 66:242+. N. '85.

Protecting ourselves against AIDS. Rodale, R. Prevention. 37:17-18+. D. '85.

The gay dilemma. Meredith, Nikki. Psychology Today. 18:56-62. Ja. '84.

*Responding to the psychological crisis of AIDS. Morin, Stephen F. and Batchelor, Walter F. Public Health Reports. 99:4-9. Ja./F. '84.

Intravenous drug users and acquired immune deficiency syndrome. Ginsberg, Harold M. Public Health Reports. 99:206-11. Mr./Ap. '84.

Can kids catch AIDS in school? Kaplan, H. Redbook. 166:12. F. '86.

Is there death after sex? Colen, B. D. Rolling Stone. p. 17. F. 3, '83.

Death in the family. Van Gelder, L. Rolling Stone. pp.18-20+. F. 3, '83.

The plague years. Black, David. Rolling Stone. I:48-50+. Mr. 28, '85; II: 35-6+. Ap. 25, '85.

The epidemiology of AIDS: current status and future prospects. Science. pp. 1352-7. S. 27, '85.

AIDS trends: projections from limited data. Norman, Colin. Science. pp. 1018-21. N. 29, '85.

Politics and science clash on African AIDS. Norman, Colin. Science. pp.1140-2. D. 6, '85.

Congress likely to halt shrinkage in AIDS funds. Norman, Colin. Science. pp. 1364-5. Mr. 21, '86.

AIDS-related brain damage unexplained. Barnes, Deborah M. Science. pp. 1091-3. My. 30, '86.

*Grim projections for AIDS epidemic. Barnes, Deborah M. Science. pp. 1589-90. Je. 27, '86.

AIDS in the blood. Scientific American. 251:89+. S. '84.

Bad blood? Scientific American. 253:78-79. D. '85.

The immune system in AIDS. Laurence, Jeffrey. Scientific American. 253:84-93. D. '85.

AIDS: a spreading scourge. Wallis, Claudia. Time. 126:50-1. Ag. 5, '85.

The new untouchables. Thomas, E. Time. 126:24-6. S. 23, '85.

A scourge spreads panic. Serrill, M. S. Time. 126:50-2. O. 28, '85.

Donating blood for yourself. Wallis, Claudia. Time. 127:63. Jl. 21, '86.

AIDS goes to court [victims sue to stop discrimination]. Lacayo, R. Time. 128:73. D. 8, '86.

*Surgeon general's report on acquired immune deficiency syndrome. U. S. Department of Health and Human Services. '86.

Rock Hudson AIDS case sends a message. U. S. News & World Report. 99:12. Ag. 5, '85.

Africa's latest torment: AIDS. U. S. News & World Report. 99:8. D. 23, '85.

The rivalry to defeat AIDS. Carey, Joseph. U. S. News & World Report. 100:67–8. Ja. 13, '86.

AIDS triggers painful legal battles. Gest, T. U. S. News & World Report. 100:69–70. S. 29, '86.

AIDS: at the dawn of fear [special section; with editorial comment by Morton B. Zuckerman]. U. S. News & World Report. 102:60–70,76. Ja. 12, '87.

Many firms fire AIDS victims, citing health risk to co-workers. Wall Street Journal. p. 21. Ag. 12, '85.

Employers and insurers have reason to fear expensive epidemic. Wall Street Journal. p. 1. O. 18, '85.

Tenfold increase in cases of AIDS is expected by 1991, . . . 179,000 deaths within that time period. Wall Street Journal. p. 10. Je. 13, '86.

AIDS has spread 'almost everywhere' in Africa, Zaire doctor tells parley. Wall Street Journal. p. 63. Je. 24, '86.

AIDS researchers urge refinements to blood testing, more drug studies. Wall Street Journal. p. 38. Je. 25, '86.

Haitians and AIDS. Washington Post. p. A22. Ap. 13, '85.

AIDS uncertainties causing change in politics on blood transfusions. Engel, Margaret. Washington Post. p. A16. Ja. 10, '86.

Half of gays carry AIDS antibody in San Francisco's neighborhood. Berg, Paul. Washington Post. p. WH5. Ja. 29, '86.

AIDS vaccine testing could start in 1988. Washington Post. p. 147. My. 7, '86.

Ethics and AIDS. Allen, G. World Press Review. 33:53. F. '86.